# Connective Tissue Diseases

This book is not intended to replace the services of a licensed physician. Any application of the recommendations set forth in the following pages is at the reader's discretion and sole risk. A major goal of this book is to explain the important relationship between correct nutrition and good health, but also to offer safe natural treatment solutions to the chronically ill connective tissue disease patient. Holistic therapy focuses on the prevention of new symptoms and improving existing symptoms with natural substances. All life-threatening situations must be treated by the attending physician.



First printing: 2002
Second printing 2003

Cover design by Hannelore Helbing-Sheafe, Ph.D.


ISBN: 1-59109-980-3

To order additional copies, please contact us.
BookSurge, LLC
www.booksurge.com
1-866-308-6235
orders@booksurge.com

# Connective Tissue Diseases
# Holistic Therapy Options

Sjoegren's Syndrome
Systemic Sclerosis—Scleroderma
Systemic Lupus Erythematosus
Discoid Lupus Erythematosus
Secondary and Primary Raynaud's phenomenon
Raynaud's Disease
Polymyositis—Dermatomyositis
Mixed Connective Tissue Disease

---

Hannelore Helbing-Sheafe, Ph.D.

Huckleberry Hill Press
1547-101st. Ave. S.W.
Olympia, WA 98512-1054

2003

# Connective Tissue Diseases

# Table of Contents


| | |
|---|---|
| Author's words | xi |
| My reason for writing this book | xv |
| How can this book be of help? | xvii |
| How to use this book... | xix |
| Preface | xxv |
| Holistic therapy options—a safe alternative | xxvii |
| Chapter I | 1 |
| A patient's story | 1 |
| Discussion of symptoms | 3 |
| Chapter II | 15 |
| The Connective Tissue Diseases | 15 |
| Sjoegren's Syndrome | 15 |
| Discussion of holistic therapy options | 23 |
| Systemic Sclerosis (Scleroderma) | 29 |
| Localized Scleroderma | 31 |
| Discussion of holistic therapy options | 39 |
| Goals of holistic therapy for the Scleroderma patient | 43 |
| How certain nutrients and herbs can help the Scleroderma patient and other connective tissue disease. patients | 51 |
| Systemic Lupus Erythematosus (SLE) | 55 |
| Discoid (cutaneous) Lupus Erythematosus (DLE) | 55 |
| Drug induced Lupus and Neonatal Lupus | 55 |
| Discussion of holistic therapy options | 67 |
| Suggested nutrient supplementation program for SLE and DLE Lupus patients | 75 |
| The importance of using the right fats | 85 |
| Special Kidney Section | 87 |
| Holistic therapy for kidney and urinary tract problems | 87 |
| Vasculitis in Lupus Erythematosus | 93 |
| Discussion of holistic therapy options for the Lupus patient | 97 |
| Primary and Secondary Raynaud's phenomenon | 99 |

and Raynaud's disease 99
Discussion of holistic therapy options for
Raynaud's phenomenon and disease 109
Raynaud's disease 113
Polymyositis—Dermatomyositis 115
Inclusion Myositis—Juvenile Myositis
(All are "Inflammatory Myopathies") 121
Discussion of holistic therapy options
for the Myositis patient 125
Mixed Connective Tissue Disease 129
Fibromyalgia
Chapter III 131
Discussion of Holistic Therapy Options
Why nutrition instead of medicine? 131
Holistic therapy options
A discussion of essential connective tissue
nutrients and how they can be of help 133
Holistic therapy options
Natural antibiotic substances 137
Holistic therapy options
Natural Substances to fight Infections and
Inflammations
How to fight back with natural substances 139
Holistic therapy options
How to strengthen the immune system 141
Holistic therapy options
Natural anti-inflammatory and pain-reducing
substances 143
Holistic Therapy Options
Natural pain fighters for bones, muscles,
ligaments, tendons, lymph system and glands 147
Discussion of holistic therapy options
The role of ascorbic acid in Connective Tissue
Diseases (Collagen Diseases), Rheumatoid
Arthritis, Osteoarthritis and Rheumatism 151
Holistic Therapy Options

Natural Vasodilators Especially important for patients with Raynaud's phenomenon or Raynaud's disease who are at risk for gangrene, stroke or suffering from high blood pressure 153
Holistic Therapy Options
Natural Antioxidants 159
Holistic Therapy Options
Natural therapy for skin conditions 161
Holistic Therapy Options
Natural Insomnia Fighters
Natural Tranquilizers and Sedatives 165
Holistic Therapy Options
Glandular nutrients for the C.T.D. patient 167
Holistic Therapy Options
To counteract stress and calm the body 169
Holistic Therapy Options
Nutrients and herbs for the mind and brain tissues 171
Holistic Therapy Options
For spinal nerves, bones, ligaments, tendons, muscles and synovial membranes 173
Holistic Therapy Options
Neurology 177
Holistic Therapy Options
Urinary system problems 179
Holistic Therapy Options
Preventive nutrients for cancer and radiation damage 181
Holistic Therapy Options
Eye and vision problems 185
Holistic therapy options
For patients who have trouble expelling mucus 189
Holistic Therapy Options
Prevention and treatment of Cardiovascular problems in the C.T.D. patient 191
Discussion of Holistic Therapy Options
Stroke prevention 193
Holistic Therapy Options

Natural Candida Fighters to help the C.T.D. Patient 195
Chapter IV 197
What patients need to know about certain supplements before beginning a holistic program and how and why these supplements work 197
Author's Personal Supplement Program used for the completely natural treatment of Mixed Connective Tissue Disease with symptoms of SLE, Sjoegren's and Raynaud's phenomenon 209
Chapter V 213
What is Connective Tissue? 213
What is Collagen?
And why is Ascorbic Acid so important? 227

Chapter VI 229
A private study involving eleven connective tissue disease patients 229
The following subjects were covered in the study:
Study results 231
Progress report 234
Index 239
Suggested Reading 257

# Author's words

A very sick patient said: "I'm the only expert in my disease, because only I know all the different kinds of pain, only I feel and experience everything that has gone wrong with my body. No doctor could know or understand what I know about me!"

Connective tissue diseases produce such a complex set of symptoms that it often takes years, before a patient is diagnosed correctly. But even then physicians cannot be certain, if the patient has only Lupus, only Raynaud's, only Sjoegren's Syndrome, only Scleroderma or all of them together because he/she can have several symptoms from each of them. Until the diagnosis is made, many patients suffer not only from their long-standing health problems but also from the indifference of family, friends and physicians since all are uncomfortable with the chronically ill individual.

The patient with connective tissue disease has varying and ever changing problems all the time. One day it can be a vasospasm which shuts down circulation into a leg or foot making it ice cold and extremely painful. The next day there could be cramping of abdominal muscles. And on another day there could be a sudden spasm of the esophagus, or a severe pain radiating from the stomach to the jaw bone or into the upper back. On still another day the patient awakens with a fever high enough to cause concern and of course, misery. The fever days may also produce sickening headaches, or a sore stomach, bloating and other digestive problems. There may be immense pressure in the lower back of the skull, which makes walking or any movement or vibration painful and causes simultaneous pressure on the eyes and a feeling of dizziness. The neck muscles might be so taut, that no amount of stretching will release the tension. There may be days, when the kidneys hurt and fluid retention becomes a problem. Such is the life of these unfortunate souls! ***Granted, there are some predictable symptoms for each of the connective tissue diseases, which can be verified by lab tests. But, on the other hand and to the frustration of doctor and patient alike, a "positive" does not always mean that the person tested has this problem, and "negative" does not always mean that the patient doesn't have a problem. Some physicians write off patients with multi-symptoms as "hypochondriacs" or simply refer them to a psychiatric counselor. This action shames the patient. The symptoms are real; the disease is real, so how could a psychiatrist be of use?

Modern medicine has lost touch with the true meaning of "healing". Patients "take a number" in the multi-physician clinic. Patients are "statistics", inhuman numbers. And patients know what is missing in their treatment. They know when compassion, caring and paying attention to details are missing. They are hurt, frustrated, angry, disappointed, hopeless and faceless people, who just want somebody to put an arm around them and say: "I am here for you. We will get to the bottom of this. Be patient and we will work this out together!" That is what they want and need to hear and need to feel. ***Many family members don't understand, just how unbearably miserable this situation is for a patient with connective tissue disease because they don't feel the pain, and they don't want to listen anymore. They just want to shut out the daily reports of misery. ***I want to send this message to the fathers, mothers, sisters and brothers, husbands and wives, doctors and nurses: "Be kind to this person. You might have even said things like "God, every day she/he has a different pain or complaint!" Please, don't shame them; don't strip away their dignity by ignoring them or making fun of them, or worse... sending them to a psychiatrist, because you don't want to listen anymore!" Patients with connective tissue disease have a tough enough time as it is. They don't need extra stress in their lives. All they need is love and understanding, and that will go a long way towards helping this person to be well.

The reader will find natural and safe solutions in this book, which can lead to a much healthier and happier life. *** What each patient must know is this: "You have to take total responsibility for your own well-being. Nobody else can do that for you!" And, if you are under medical care and on medication at this time; "please, do not interpret this book to mean, that you should stop your current treatment. Do not forfeit valuable medical crisis care!" But, I hope that you will share the information with your medical counselor and that you and he will have the courage, to give holistic options a really fair try. This can only be accomplished, if sufficient time and correct nutrient or herbal dosages are allowed to do their work and improve your health

Connective tissue diseases are nutrient deficiency diseases, which become especially active during or after prolonged and acute mental, physical or chemical stress. Patients should know that there is hope and positive results can be achieved, once a commitment has been made. Please, remember this affirmation and use it often each day:

"Each cell of my body is filled with God's healing energy!"

# My reason for writing this book

I arrived in San Diego, California in 1959, a brand-new immigrant from Germany. Trying to adjust to a totally different language, being homesick, eating and drinking very different foods and just trying to adjust to my new country caused considerable stress. I began to experience sore throats, swollen glands, fevers and fatigue. The attending physician made a hasty diagnosis of "infectious mononucleosis" without using lab tests and prescribed large amounts of penicillin. My immediate reaction to penicillin was this:

- Always extremely tight muscles
- Colic-type intestinal pains due to the destruction of beneficial intestinal flora and resulting breakdown of normal bowel health. These pains eventually became so severe, that my physician prescribed morphine.

  In the months and years following high penicillin treatment I experienced these symptoms:
- Mood changes
- Phobias (due to B-vitamin deficiencies)
- Skin changes; Vitiligo and a plantar wart developed.
- Toe and finger nails began to develop ridges
- Rapid development of cavities. Several teeth were lost within 5 years after the penicillin treatment.

- Weight problem developed due to now malfunctioning thyroid and adrenal glands
- General health poor

  These symptoms were caused by substantial nutritional problems due to malfunctioning bowels and subsequent undernourishment.

Frequent visits to my medical counselor were frustrating and unsuccessful. Because of my list of consistent complaints I was put into the category of undesirable, unstable patients, the kind of patients most doctors don't know what to do with and therefore write off as "neurotic". And yes, my doctor told me at one point: "Go home and figure out what your problems are there because I don't know!" ***In my search for an answer I began to experiment with many different natural food supplements. Eventually I learned what and how much of it could make me feel better. In 1976 my husband was struck down with a major heart attack. He survived, but never worked again. I became his sole caregiver until he passed away in 1992. These years of unrelenting stress weakened my immune system even further. In 1988 I suffered my first breakdown with connective tissue disease...*** Today I am healthier. My illness gave me a powerful motivation to help myself with holistic therapy and natural substances and to share my research with others, so they too can feel better. And that is why I wrote this book. ***I suggest that patients use daily positive affirmations to reinforce the healing process and to regain control. Most of all they must know that they can change the direction of their illness by being informed and giving their body important support through the use of safe and natural substances.

Words and thoughts are powerful!

Therefore, if I accept that I am chronically ill, then I will never be well again!

# How can this book be of help?

- It lets patients learn what symptoms they have in common with other connective tissue disease patients. This eases the isolation many patients feel, because they previously felt misunderstood and alone.
- It provides information what types of nutrients, herbs or other natural substances can be used to restore specific body tissues to normal function, such as bone tissue, tendons, ligaments, muscles, membranes or blood vessels. Knowing that something can be done increases a patient's hope of regaining quality of life and not to be considered a totally hopeless case.
- It teaches how to use "selective nutrient support" to interrupt or prevent arterial spasms which otherwise could lead to ulceration, gangrene and loss of limbs or life. Now the patient can take charge. Knowledge makes it easier to take responsibility for one's own health.
- It teaches how to use "selective nutrient support" to rebuild collagen and restore the integrity of damaged or malfunctioning connective tissue. It gives patients hope knowing that the illness can be modified and possibly reversed and stabilized.
- It teaches how to use "selective nutrient support" to

prevent, reduce or completely eliminate pain. Any pain reduction is valuable, because it allows the body to relax, to sleep better and allow body cells to do their repair work.

- It teaches how to use "selective nutrient therapy" to increase lubrication fluids for the eyes (e.g. dry eye in Sjoegren's Syndrome) and other membranes, such as the inside of the mouth and vaginal tissues. Again, just knowing that something can be done to improve symptoms sets in motion positive, helpful feelings, which aid the healing process.
- It teaches how to use "selective nutrient support" or other holistic therapy which addresses other common symptoms, such as impaired circulation, slow thinking, forgetfulness, numbness, tingling, and coldness of limbs.

# How to use this book

A detailed "table of contents" gives the reader instant access to specific points of interest. Equally, a substantial "index" provides further valuable help in finding those subjects, which are of personal interest to the individual.

The index is followed by a "Suggested Reading List" of thirty-one authors, some famous as writers and researchers in the holistic field, for instance Linus Pauling. This list represents a large percentage of my mental tutors, whose knowledge I have used and built upon to help myself and others throughout my 30 year career as a holistic practitioner, researcher and writer.

Chapter I. A patient's story—lists specific symptoms, information about which organs and other body structures can be involved, the importance of annual blood tests, hair analysis and using Reflexology, Iridology and other methods of holistic testing. The listing of symptoms allows patients to compare and mark those they have experienced.

Chapter II—Connective tissue diseases

- Sjoegren's Syndrome symptoms; its connection to other forms of connective tissue diseases; current medical treatment and safe holistic treatment options

- Scleroderma (Systemic Sclerosis), symptoms; current medical treatment and safe holistic treatment options
- Systemic Lupus Erythematosus (SLE), Discoid Lupus Erythematosus (DLE), Neonatal and drug-induced Lupus, symptoms; current medical treatment and safe holistic treatment options
- Vasculitis in Lupus, symptoms; holistic treatment options; current medical treatment and safe holistic treatment options
- Primary and Secondary Raynaud's phenomenon and Raynaud's disease symptoms; current medical treatment and safe holistic therapy options
- Polymyositis and Dermatomyositis, symptoms; current medical treatment and safe holistic therapy options
- Mixed connective tissue disease and Fibromyalgia—brief explanation and safe holistic therapy options

Chapter III—Holistic therapy options

Explains the use and value of specific nutrients, single herbs or herbal combinations and other natural substances for all forms of connective tissue disease symptoms.

Provides lists of

- Natural antibiotics for viral and bacterial infections
- Natural anti-fungal remedies to fight Candida and other fungal infections
- Natural anti-inflammatory and pain fighting substances
- Natural vasodilators
- Natural substances to fight skin problems
- Natural tranquilizers and sedatives
- Natural substances for mental symptoms
- Natural substances for kidney and bladder problems
- Natural substances for cardiovascular problems
- Natural substances for neurological problems
- Natural substances for eye problems

Chapter IV—Guidelines to supplementation program

How much and why certain natural substances work well

Chapter V—Provides information about connective tissue,

collagen production and why ascorbic acid (vitamin C) plays such an important role in the holistic therapy management of connective tissue disease and its multiple symptoms and offers special information about sub-scurvy and scurvy symptoms and its relationship to connective tissue disease.

Chapter VI—Lists results of a private study of 11 patients diagnosed with connective tissue disease. The study revealed startling results about similar medical histories of the participants.

To my daughters Susanne, Karen and Christa

# Preface

Lupus, Vasculitis in Lupus, Scleroderma, and Raynaud's disease, Raynaud's phenomenon, Polymyositis, Dermatomyositis and Sjoegren's Syndrome are connective tissue diseases. They belong to the large family of arthritis-type illnesses. ***A 1995 government publication stated that between 35 and 40 million Americans are afflicted by arthritis. Now, in 2003, this number is dramatically higher. ***The accepted medical approach follows well established guidelines. However, treatment is basically for pain and infections only. Booklets available from the American Arthritis Foundation offer very little help beyond explaining symptoms, exercise programs and available drug treatment. Many patients suffer from a variety of symptoms for many years before a clear diagnosis can be made by their physician because many of their symptoms resemble those of other illnesses. Obviously the uncertainty puts patients under great stress. ***Once diagnosed and receiving medication, new problems arise. The medications have mild to sometimes very severe side effects, adding new physical stress to a body already stressed beyond tolerance. *** Sadly most patients do not expect to be well again and this negative belief system further weakens their bodies. They are willing in most cases to bargain just for pain relief, so they can make it through another day. But pain medication creates an illusion of being better, while the actual illness progresses unhindered.

# Holistic therapy options—a safe alternative

Patients have a right to know about safe alternatives. The author was diagnosed in 1988 with "mixed connective tissue disease". This diagnostic term is used, when a patient experiences overlapping symptoms of several types of connective tissue diseases. In this case symptoms of Raynaud's phenomenon, Sjoegren's, Scleroderma and Lupus were experienced. ***The most impressive improvement of symptoms in the author's case was achieved with holistic treatment, when the beginning stages of "gangrene" were reversed and the affected foot and leg regained normal circulation. This was accomplished, after the affected limb was shown to the attending physician who stated "that very little could be done to stop gangrene and that he had seen several patients with Raynaud's phenomenon who had already lost digits". ***How was the reversal of gangrene accomplished? By studying the effects of nutrition on human body cells, finding important links between certain nutritional deficiencies and resulting disease and then using this knowledge to reverse the disease process. Many different dosages of vitamins, minerals, trace elements, different herbal medicines and a variety of specialty nutrients were tried, until results began to appear. Now, 15 years after the initial diagnosis, the author is almost fully productive. Some of the symptoms are gone completely, others are greatly diminished. Mind and body are in much better shape than in 1988. However, a few symptoms can recur when supplement therapy is relaxed (not enough or not consistently), when physical activity is grossly overdone (e.g. shoveling snow or spading a garden for hours), or when sudden sugar cravings lead to excessive carbohydrate intake and cause a flare-up of fungal infections. Eating too much meat also causes flare-ups because excessive protein intake makes the body too acid and inflammation follows. ***Heavy sugar use, even in the form of fruit or fruit juices, feeds the ravenous yeast fungus. And seemingly harmless things like grapes (natural yeast on skins), wine, beer, soy sauce, mushrooms, yeast breads and crackers, pizza, certain cheeses and favorite spaghetti sauces with mushrooms can still bring on a new round of shortness of breath, severe vice-like pain, spiking fevers, skin rashes, flu-like symptoms and much pain. *** Commercially sold meats contain substantial antibiotic traces. The accumulative effect of using such products can continuously activate the yeast fungus and start a relapse. These foods should be avoided. Many patients experience repeated Candida infections because they take birth control pills or are on hormone replacement therapy. Too much sun, too much work, too much acid food, too much sugar, too many yeast products, being exposed to mold and mildew—all these are "red flags" for patients with fungal problems. Why is it important to explore the possible presence of Candida or any of the other yeast fungi in a patient's body? Please read on. ***A private study of eleven patients (chapter VI), diagnosed with one or more of the connective tissue diseases, revealed that all had one thing in common: Overuse of antibiotics in earlier years and resulting Candida and other fungal infections later in life. Fungal infections can be life threatening when unchecked and are capable of infiltrating major body organs, including the brain. The reader is advised to request tests for the presence of yeast fungi. Both medical and naturopathic physicians can order this test for you. If the result comes back "positive" look up chapter III, which lists natural and safe anti-fungal substances.

The following information is of great importance to all patients: Please, understand and always remember that a body under stress from disease cannot assimilate enough nutrients from a normal diet and will continue to experience severe nutrient deficiencies, unless high-potency vitamin and mineral supplements are used consistently to support the nutritional needs of sick individuals.

# Chapter I
## A patient's story

It was summer 1988. My ailing husband leaned back in his recliner. My daughter Christa retired to her room and I was washing dishes. Suddenly a strange cold feeling came over me. The left half of my face began to feel numb. I felt as if the airway in the left nostril was constricted and I couldn't get air through it. Then my tongue began to feel numb. I could not swallow saliva. This was followed quickly by a sensation of heaviness, coldness and numbness in the left arm and hand. My thoughts began to slow. Thoughts and body seemed to be in slow motion. My left buttock suddenly felt very cold. I had the distinct feeling that ice water was running through this tissue. This was followed by a terribly painful cold feeling in my left lower leg, then ankle and foot. ***At this point I was not only very frightened, but believed I was having a stroke. But then rational thinking returned and let me realize, that I couldn't think clearly if I were having a stroke. To reinforce that thought process, my right side began to grow numb also. However, this side was not affected as severely as the left. But what in God's name had happened to me? ***I fought desperately to maintain control; to stop this horrible feeling from going any further. All I knew was that some internal switch had malfunctioned and peripheral blood circulation was almost completely shut down. My left arm hung heavy by my side. My left leg was so cold and numb that I could not feel my foot at all. Nor could I feel my lip or nose on the left side of my face. ***This was my first introduction to C.T.D. (connective tissue disease). It took many weeks, before some of the pain and coldness subsided. Many more episodes followed, before I slowly began to learn and understand what was happening and initially self-diagnosed my problem. Later I went to see a medical physician who concluded, that some of my symptoms were those of "Raynaud's phenomenon". I was also told that I had "mixed connective tissue disease". ***Even today, 15 years later, milder attacks can occur. Heavy throbbing music coming from passing cars, the powerful high pitched hour-long whine of a neighbor's riding mower, vibrations from a hand held weed eater, chain saw or my truck's engine, or ear piercing screams from a child—they all can prompt an attack. These attacks are milder now and work through my system much more quickly because of skills learned to cope with the problem. I still feel annoying pains in my finger tips when during a relapse I accidentally touch a metal button on my jacket and the overly sensitive nerves in the fingers register the slightest temperature change and send pain signals. Playing my string instruments now is sometimes a little painful, but no longer totally impossible. Progress has been made! ***The following pages list symptoms by categories. This allows the reader the opportunity to compare and mark off those symptoms which may have been experienced or are still present. It seems strange, that so many different body tissues can be affected, yet it is true. It can happen. ***Based on the observation of my own symptoms and the results of the study of eleven other patients diagnosed with C.T.D the following symptoms were experienced by all in various degrees.

# Discussion of symptoms

## Head

- Strong pressure in lower back of skull; sometimes so strong, that each step or each vibration causes immediate discomfort, often severe pain
- Heavy burning feeling behind the eyes
- Scalp muscles contracted; very tender to touch
- Forehead muscles contract and twitch; feel tight
- Tissue two inches from hair line—severe spasms
- Trouble swallowing; slowness
- Lack of feeling in throat and esophagus; actually feels cold inside when food/drink passes through; spasms of esophagus
- Feeling of a steel band around skull; pressure inward

## Teeth

- Pain when drinking cool or cold liquids
- Continuing decay in spite of good dental hygiene
- Gum disease developing; bleeding; pain
- After new dental fillings constant acid tasting excessive saliva discharges
- Vibration from drilling brings on new Raynaud's phenomenon attack
- Stretching of jaw during dental procedure produced dizziness, loss of balance, loss of feelings in the legs, headaches and hissing sounds in the ears. This indicates involvement of connective tissue in the temporal-mandibular joints.
- Pain felt in all teeth much of the time

## Ears

- Feeling of fullness and pressure
- Ears burn

- Hissing sounds much of the time, especially after carbohydrate consumption.
- Hissing sounds worse when in reclined or semi-reclined position
- Pressure in ears; occasional shooting pain

## Eyes

- Pressure in eye ball
- Heaviness of lid; feeling of drooping
- Floaters, especially after sugar binges
- Eyes hurt after computer work
- Eyes feel gritty and dry
- Frequent deep ache in eye ball
- Seeing stars or light flashes when turning head quickly
- Painful, takes effort to focus

## Throat

- Deep throat pain in area of Adam's apple
- Pain when swallowing cold liquid or food

## Jaws

- Frequent swelling of lymph nodes
- Frequent swelling and inflammation of Parotid glands
- Jawbones very tight during active attack. Feeling of rigidity in facial bones and muscles

## Mouth

- Painless bumps inside mouth
- Tissue feels inflamed, irritated
- Gum tissue swollen, bleeds easily
- Frequent very dry mouth (Sjoegren's Syndrome)
- Occasional sudden and profuse saliva production
- During active Raynaud's phenomenon attack: roof of mouth hurts when drinking cool or cold liquids. This is felt as a deep strong ache especially in the tonsil area and

the roof of the mouth

- Tongue burns
- Tongue is swollen

## Spine

- Extreme pain felt in tissue in thoracic spine from T6 through T8Pain radiating from T6 to 10th rib
- Pain radiating from T7 to scapulae
- Deep pain in area T2 through T5
- Tissue from T12 through L2 is contracted and cannot be stretched
- Pain is felt in all spinal muscles during active C.T.D episodes. Difficulty leaning against toilet tank, back of chair or to lie flat

## Bones, muscles, tendons and ligaments

- Patients in the study reported that for many years preceding the acute onset of their illness they all suffered from tight muscles, tendons and ligaments in many different body areas. Stretching did not help. Some relief was obtained from walking.
- Outer foot and ankle muscles so weak that it cannot hold up patient or allowed walking only on outside of foot
- Weakness in one or both wrists. Slightest turning motion causes extreme pain
- Muscles of one or both feet feel contracted
- Hardened muscle tissue areas found in arms and legs which cannot be massaged away (Sjoegren's syndrome)
- Deep tissue pain in upper abdominal muscles, sometimes spasms and extreme tightening
- Deep tissue pain at tip of sternum, especially after exertion
- Extreme tightness around lower rib cage, spanning from one side of the spine around lower ribs to other side of
- spine, producing a feeling of a steel band tightening rib cage. Effects breathing and causes severe pain

- Sternocleidomastoid muscle on both sides contracted from skull to collar bone. Difficulty turning head
- Hamstring muscle—deep pain; feeling of contracting
- Gracilis muscle; deep pain and contracted
- Sciatic nerve involvement; causes deep pain in pelvis and legs and contracture of surrounding muscle tissue
- Skull sutures; misalignment causing severe cranial pressure
- Masseter (chewing muscle); inability to move jawbones normally; pain chewing. Usually accompanied by swollen Parotid glands
- Lateral neck muscle spasms
- All muscular tissues of skull contracted
- Always sore muscles, fascia and tendons

## Skin, nails and hair

- Rashes on arms
- Rashes on face
- Yeast rashes come and go, appear instantly after sugar use or exposure to mildew, mold, yeast and fermented products
- Vitiligo was reported in some patients
- During relapse episodes skin of hands, feet, lower arms and face show bluish-purple color
- Blotchy yellow-brown spots on hands and arms
- Hangnails
- Build-up of calluses on heels
- Bronze-colored areas in groin, underarms, face or neck
- Skin extremely sore to touch during relapse episodes. Clothing may be too irritating.
- Dry skin
- Capillary damage showing on face and ankles
- Nose tip tissue has changed. Now bumpy and indentations
- Nose tip swells
- Yeast irritation constant in vaginal area and groin, ranging

from annoying to very severe, accompanied by severe itching.
- Weight gain in abdominal tissue; development of skin flab

## Fingers

- Stiff and painful
- Skin blanched
- Extremely sensitive to hot and cold
- Parched and shriveled look
- Pale skin color at times, other times bluish
- Fatty swollen looking pads on top of fingers during active Raynaud's episodes

## Hands and arms

- Tremors
- Joints extremely tender
- Muscles harden
- Heavy at times

## Toes and feet

- Toe muscles contract and are difficult to move
- In some patients early signs of "gangrene".
- Occasionally toes lock, making it difficult to walk
- Weak muscle and tendon tissues cannot hold up weight of person; foot collapses outward; person affected has to walk on outside ridge of foot
- Feet often numb
- Feet feel ice cold
- Sole of feet frequently numb
- Occasional mild tremor
- Foot muscles contract

## Sacrum

- Tissues between sacrum and L1 contracted; cannot be stretched

- Sacrum locks; cannot be stretched

## Hips

- Movement limited, feeling of extreme tightness
- During active episodes tissue of buttocks feels as if ice water runs through the blood vessels, producing an intense burning, yet ice-cold sensation
- Intense burning pain radiating from Gluteal muscles down to the center of Hamstring muscles
- Pain in hips when sitting

## Legs

- Achilles tendons and Soleus muscle contracted
- Lower leg muscles harden
- Both legs feel very tight and very heavy
- Lower legs frequently ice cold; cannot be warmed with socks or warm water. (Arterial spasms)
- Quadriceps muscles contract; cannot be stretched

## Knees

- Knee motion limited; stiffness; tightness
- Muscles tissues above knees contract

## Chest and rib cage

- Cramping and tightness in chest
- Serratus muscles contract, making breathing difficult and painful
- Pain in sternum and tip of sternum

## Collar bones

- Feeling of tightness as if being pushed inward
- Feeling of collar bones being held in unnatural position

## Facial bones

- Bones don't move freely. Muscles contract making chewing

and speaking difficult

- Entire face feels tight. Difficult to smile. (rigid, frozen facial muscles are seen in advanced Scleroderma patients)
- Facial tightness complicates dental work and results in pain in the back of the skull and neck
- Difficulty smiling

## Temple

- Throbbing
- Occasional spasms

## Skull

- Back of skull muscles contract
- Forehead muscles contract; sometimes remain rigid
- Numbness felt in scalp tissue

## Arms

- Muscles of upper arm contract
- Hardened tissue in muscles of upper arm

## Abdomen

- Deep soreness in upper abdominal region
- Upper abdominal area feels full, tight and swollen
- Occasional severe pain in esophagus when swallowing
- Lower abdomen sore occasionally

## Urinary system

- Deep pain in kidney area, radiating into abdomen
- Diminished urination during fever periods
- Some patients develop kidney stones
- Frequent urination, especially at night
- Fluid retention problems

## Reproductive system

- Chronic yeast infections

- Discharges, especially when yeast infection is active

## Respiratory system

- Lack of oxygen accompanied by extreme tightness of center of upper abdomen. This tightness is felt in all of the lower ribs and tip of sternum
- Problems with thick mucus in bronchi and/or lungs
- Voice is husky; a feeling of lack of saliva
- Sometimes shortness of breath at night because of contracted Serratus muscle, rib cage, diaphragm and upper abdominal muscles
- Hiatus hernia flare-ups

## Nervous system

- Involuntary chills
- Numbness in face, lips and nostrils
- Numbness in legs and feet
- Numbness in arms and hands
- Feeling of paralysis in throat and epiglottis
- Tongue feels numb
- Slowness of movements of legs; feeling of not being quite in control
- Slowness of finer hand movements; fingers slow to respond; strength not affected by this
- Finger tips extremely sensitive to cold, heat, rough surfaces, sharp surfaces
- Sensitivity to loud noises
- Sensitivity to strong vibrations from music, automobile or other engines
- Pain and tenderness in cerebellum area
- Feeling of bugs crawling on skin and scalp
- Sudden sharp, needle-like pains which can occur almost anywhere
- Speech sometimes slow, clumsy, uncoordinated
- Speech sometimes slow, halting; searching for words
- Tip of tongue burns

- Roof of mouth very painful when drinking cold fluids
- Mouth is very dry
- Restless sleep
- Feeling of internal coldness
- Sometimes feeling of being overheated
- Frequent itching
- Crying spells
- Rashes thought to be caused by nerves
- Occasional tremors of extremities
- Easily irritated, on edge
- Occasional numbness; whole body feels numb, scalp to feet; speech slurry; tongue, lips and nose feel numb; eye lids feel heavy and numb

### Glandular system

- Suspected adrenal burn-out
- Suspected pancreas involvement

### Mental processes

- Slowness of thought
- Split-second haziness

### Circulatory system

- Severe arterial spasms
- Shutdown of peripheral circulation to legs and arms
- Fluid retention
- High blood pressure
- Palpitations
- Facial puffiness (edema)
- Eyelids puffy (edema)
- Alternate between feeling cold and too warm
- Cramps in legs
- Frequent pain in veins of legs and groin
- Shortness of breath

## Digestive system

- Much bloating
- Problems with intestinal gas
- Sometimes loose bowels
- Pain in esophagus
- Burning sensation in esophagus
- Irritation at top of esophagus
- Severe esophageal spasms
- Occasional reflux at night
- Excessive appetite
- Yeast food, mold, mildew, fermented food causes yeast fungus to react—many digestive problems because of that
- Occasional gastritis
- Abdominal muscle spasms with digestive upset
- Diaphragm spasms, causing upset stomach. ***Stress also plays a contributing role in frequent relapses of C.T.D. The more stress, the more active the disease becomes. ***Annual complete blood tests can provide the first clues that the body is malfunctioning. By carefully comparing each test with those of previous years, patients can often detect a definite pattern and take preventive action. For instance, if there is a pattern of impaired protein digestion, then the problem must be corrected through correct nutrition. If tests reveal an alkaline system, then corrective measures must be taken. Impaired glandular function, low blood iron and the presence of Candida or other yeast fungi all of these must be corrected to achieve better health. ***Another way to detect early warning signs is an annual iridology test. This test is usually available through holistic clinics. The layers of the iris provide instant information about body tissue changes. An experienced iridology practitioner will take a special photo of a patient's eyes and then interpret any abnormalities. In the author's case a comparison of annual iridology readings revealed early problems with the digestive system and both pituitary and thyroid glands. These problems worsened

in later years. ***Other holistic diagnostic tools are hair analysis tests which can detect early signs of C.T.D. For instance hair tests can detect glandular malfunction and certainly provide information about nutrient deficiencies. In one patient such a test revealed low manganese and zinc levels. Low nutrient levels of these two nutrients have been identified in Lupus and other autoimmune diseases. A chronically low manganese level appears to predispose a patient to autoimmune diseases.

# Chapter II
# The Connective Tissue Diseases

## Sjoegren's Syndrome
## General information

Medical researchers consider Sjoegren's syndrome an incurable, lifelong auto-immune disorder. Holistic researchers on the other hand have had some success in helping such patients, by using selective nutrients to rebuild and normalize affected tissue.

Sjoegren's syndrome is divided into two basic categories:

- Primary Sjoegren's syndrome, which affects the tear producing glands of the eyes (lachrymals), the parotid and other salivary glands, and the Bartholins glands in the vagina. Many patients have enlarged parotid glands. Primary Sjoegren's syndrome occurs without other auto-immune diseases.
- Secondary Sjoegren's syndrome, which produces typical Sjoegren's syndrome symptoms in the presence of other connective tissue problems, especially Systemic Lupus Erythematosus.
- Present data suggests that up to four million Americans are affected and that the majority of patients are women.

- Sjoegren's syndrome affects all races and all ages, but occurs mostly in women past age 50.

The body's immune system cannot tell the difference between its own tissues and foreign substances. It attacks moisture producing glands. The immune system lacks its usual controls and allows white blood cells to infiltrate those glands which normally produce lubricating moisturizing fluids. The white blood cells can destroy these glands cause them to stop producing moisture.

## Common symptoms:

- Very dry eyes, a dry mouth and vaginal irritations.
- Symptoms are always constant. Some patients may have repeated attacks with intervals of remission. The illness is considered a benign, chronic inflammation.
- Tests show high levels of abnormal serum factors, both rheumatoid and antinuclear. Sjoegren's patients usually have the rheumatoid arthritis and Sicca complex
- Some patients suffer from progressive and severe oral, ocular, vaginal and skin dryness
- At least half of the patients have enlarged parotid glands
- Patients may have different symptoms. Some may have mild episodes; others experience a really serious form of the illness.

## Typical symptoms

- Fatigue is common. Patient is easily exhausted and has to rest a lot
- Hoarseness is common and makes speaking difficult
- Trouble swallowing
- Discomfort in any of the salivary glands which produce saliva for digestion and lubrication The sublingual gland is located directly underneath the tongue The parotid glands are located in the cheeks in front of the ears. The sub- maxillary gland is located in the back of the mouth
- These glands might be swollen, painful and the patient runs a fever

- The mouth may be constantly experiencing problems, such as swollen and very tender gums, easy bleeding and/ or frequent episodes of little painless bumps in the inside mouth tissues
- There can be cracks in the corner of the mouth
- A dry mouth (lack of moisture) can damage tooth enamel. Saliva fights bacteria. Without saliva bacteria can attack tooth enamel, resulting in many cavities
- Trouble talking because of dry larynx
- Eyes feel very dry, gritty, painful, burn and look red and irritated
- A thick substance can collect in the inside corner of the eye during sleep
- Eyes can be extremely sensitive to sunlight and any bright color
- There can be vision disturbances and blurriness
- Deprived of lubricating fluids eyes can develop corneal ulcers and, in some cases blindness
- The inside of the nose may be very dry and painful
- Vaginal tissues can dry out and become very irritated. Intercourse can be painful.
- Very dry skin is also reported by many patients.

## To summarize

Malfunction of the immune system causes white blood cells to invade the tear producing glands and lead to corneal ulceration. Malfunction of the salivary glands causes dryness and irritation, trouble speaking and swallowing due to a lack of lubrication. And, when the Bartholins glands in the vagina stop producing lubrication, vaginal dryness and resulting irritation cause great discomfort.

## Other problems

- Numbness and tingling (also found in other types of connective tissue disease
- There may be confusion
- Blood vessels may be involved (Vasculitis)

- Muscle weakness may be present
- The central nervous system can be involved
- Liver and pancreas involvement is possible

The American SSF (Sjoegren's Syndrome Foundation) reports, that the following organs can be affected:

- Kidneys
- Blood vessels
- Lungs
- Liver
- Pancreas
- Brain
- Stomach

Sjoegren's syndrome occurs with other types of connective tissue diseases, such as

- SLE (Systemic Lupus Erythematosus)
- Raynaud's Phenomenon
- Raynaud's disease
- Scleroderma
- Fibromyalgia

## Is the illness easily diagnosed?

The majority of patients with Sjoegren's syndrome are utterly frustrated, because their symptoms mimic many other diseases and a diagnosis is often delayed, until the disease has become quite severe. When a patient, for instance reports swollen gums or bumps inside the mouth to a physician little or no attention is being given to these symptoms. Reporting swollen and painful parotid glands, which limit eating and can radiate pain into surrounding tissues, may also not get specific attention; the general practitioner is usually not trained in recognizing Sjoegren's syndrome and may not consider these symptoms as anything unusual. This becomes a very frustrating experience for a person in pain, who is looking for answers…

A recent internet publication states the following common diagnostic procedures:

- Blood tests for unusual proteins (auto-antibodies)
- Tests to determine the degree of dryness of the eyes and mouth
- Sometimes lip biopsies are performed

## How is a definite diagnosis possible?

- It helps to know that post menopausal women are more prone to this problem than young women.
- Blood tests for the presence of auto-antibodies are helpful in providing information.
- Tissue biopsies are sometimes used to determine the presence of Sjoegren's syndrome.
- Physicians may look for swollen glands, a dry and cracked tongue, enlarged neck glands and itchy, red and irritated eyes.
- The "Schirmer Test" is sometimes used to determine the level of dryness in the eye. This test is described as placing filter paper under the eyelid to see how much tear fluid the eye produces in reaction to the irritation.

## The American Arthritis Foundation lists these tests:

- Slit lamp examination—dye is used to check the dryness of the eye
- Lip biopsy—removal of a few salivary glands from the inside lip
- Salivary function test—which measures the actual amount of saliva
- Urine test—to test kidney performance
- Chest x-rays to look for possible lung changes

## Is Sjoegren's syndrome curable?

Medical physicians think it is not. Holistic practitioners however, believe that people suffering from any connective tissue disease can be helped. Please, read the appropriate holistic recommendations in this chapter and chapter III.

## Current medical treatment

- Treatment to ease dryness and replace moisture, thus relieving discomfort
- Aspirin to reduce joint swelling, stiffness and muscle aches
- Nonsteroidal, anti-inflammatory drugs (NASAID's) to relieve same symptoms
- Steroids and immunosuppressive drugs for renal and pulmonary involvement
- Drugs which reduce the severity of the symptoms
- Referral to various specialists, such as rheumatologists, dentists and eye specialists
- Disease modifying drugs and antibiotics for infection
- For severe complications more aggressive treatment is used
- Recommendation for sun glasses to protect eyes from sun and dust
- Use of artificial tears

## What other conditions can contribute to a dry mouth?

- Aging
- Side effects of certain drugs
- Ionizing radiation
- Stress
- Smoking
- Pregnancy
- Cancer
- Other autoimmune disorders
- High blood pressure
- Diabetes

## Dry mouth can also occur as a result of either of the following:

- Side effect of using diuretics
- Side effect of high blood pressure medication

- Side effect of anti-depressant medication
- Side effect of chemotherapy
- Side effect of antihistamine medication
- Side effect of antibiotic medication
- Dry mouth, often seen in the elderly, can severely affect eating, speech, taste and oral health and certainly can have a pronounced psychological impact on the patient.

# Discussion of holistic therapy options

## What alternative treatment options are available?

### Dry mouth—Holistic therapy options

- SALIX, a saliva substitute, provides relief from dry mouth. This natural medicine works by stimulating the salivary glands. The manufacturers suggest that patients with dry mouth (xerostomia) avoid using candies or lozenges, since they contain sugars and acids which further destroy tooth enamel already weakened or damaged by the lack of saliva.
- Ascorbic acid (vitamin C): improves saliva production. Recommendation: 1/8 teaspoon ascorbic acid powder mixed into medium glass of water. Patient takes a little sip every one half hour, holds it in the mouth for 20 seconds, then swallows. This is followed by rinsing the mouth with clear water to remove acid residue from ascorbic acid.
- Zinc picolinate: this nutrient improves taste sensations, especially in the elderly.
- CoenzymeQ10 helps to improve gum health and stimulates saliva production. Q10 spray under the tongue is best.

- To avoid further enamel breakdown, natural toothpastes containing naturally occurring safe fluoride should be used daily.
- Holistic practitioners frown on the use of any refined sugar products because of their acid reaction inside the mouth.
- Sugar free natural chewing gum or candy also help to stimulate saliva flow
- Tea tree oil toothpicks stimulate saliva production
- If severe mouth pain prevents the patient from eating or if extreme dryness is present: liquid nutritional formulas can be used. These are available in all health food stores

## Dry eyes—holistic therapy options

- B6: (pyridoxine) 100 mg 3 x daily with meals
- Natural tears: available in health food stores
- Ascorbic acid: 5,000—8,000 mg daily taken in several dosages Ascorbic acid as a nutrient is important in the normal function of the tear ducts. It influences the maintenance of proper fluid consistency and is therefore of great help in restoring normal tear production and subsequent irrigation of the eye. Blurred vision caused by Sjoegren's syndrome also benefits from high ascorbic acid therapy. It plays a role in diabetic retinopathy and is needed along with vitamin E d-alpha tocopherol.

Researchers found that a normal eye has a higher ascorbic acid level than that of blood or other body tissues, and that an acute or chronic ascorbic acid deficiency can severely affect the eyes. The following figures represent ascorbic acid levels in various tissues: 20 found in the retina; 30 found in the cornea; 30 found in the lens; 50-90 found in the corneal epithelium. ***Chronic ascorbic acid deficiencies are found in auto-immune diseases. They must be corrected to restore tissue function.

## Dry nose membranes, hoarseness and irritated bronchial tissue—Holistic therapy options

- A humidifier will provide moisture and helps to relieve above problems
- Slippery Elm lozenges: These, chewed slowly and allowed to dissolve, coat the vocal cords and esophagus with a very thin slippery lubricant, which can ease the pain of hoarseness and a sore mouth or throat.
- Chinese herbal medicine uses Alfalfa tablets to relieve hoarseness
- European homeopathic physicians recommend chewing honey comb to relieve hoarseness as well as irritated bronchial tubes
- Drinking lots of water to relieve hoarseness and internal dryness cannot be stressed enough. Please, do not use distilled water.

## Dry vaginal tissues—Holistic therapy options

Natural products are available in all health food stores. In post-menopausal women vaginal dryness occurs very frequently and causes all kinds of problems. Whether this condition is caused by glandular changes or not, holistic practitioners have long ago identified vitamin E as a necessary nutrient for maintaining normal vaginal lubrication. Vitamin E is taken in daily dosages ranging from 400 IU to 1200 IU. However, patients with high blood pressure and a history of rheumatic fever are limited to dosages below 100 IU.

Some patients have successfully used one tablespoon of expeller pressed Almond oil to which one 400 IU capsule of vitamin E d-alpha has been added. The oils are mixed and applied to the vaginal tissue with a cotton ball.

## Oral ulcers, ulcers of the lips and tongue and thirst—Holistic therapy options

- Tissue changes occurring in Sjoegren's can lead to a loss

of taste or abnormal taste sensations. The mineral nutrient zinc will help to normalize taste sensations

- Thirst and fluid retention are common symptoms. These can be caused by mineral deficiencies. Recommended are a diet high in fruit and vegetables, drinking eight glasses of water daily and avoiding high sodium foods.
- Patients with sore lips or cracks in the corner of their mouth: Holistic researchers have identified these tissue problems as a B-vitamin deficiency. The normal diet does not provide enough B vitamins. A high potency B-vitamin supplement plus daily use of Brewer's yeast, wheat germ and whole grain food are of great help in this matter
- If dryness of the mouth is so severe, that the patient cannot eat because of ulceration or pain, then wholesome natural liquid formulas must be substituted.
- For dry mouth: one quarter of a teaspoon of ascorbic acid powder stirred into a medium size glass of water. Rinse with this several times daily. It is important to irrigate all parts of the mouth, followed by drinking the solution for further nutritional support (e.g. dry eye). Ascorbic acid also plays an important role as a natural antiseptic and is very effective against bacteria in the mouth. The mouth should then be rinsed with clear water to remove acid residues from the tooth enamel.

## For the patient with kidney or lung involvement—Holistic therapy options

- Very important: daily irrigation with at least eight glasses of quality drinking water (no distilled)
- Helpful: B6 and magnesium supplement to support the kidneys
- Use of homeopathic herbal tinctures for kidney or lung support. These are available in all health food stores.
- CoenzymeQ10: a cellular nutrient important for normalizing cell growth and to aid affected tissues. Japanese and European physicians recommend pharmaceutical

dosages of 400 mg daily.

- To minimize acidity : Recommended is a diet high in fruit, vegetables and plenty of drinking water to encourage normal lubrication and to prevent mucus from becoming thick and sticky.

## For the Sjoegren's patient with dry skin—Holistic therapy options

- Ascorbic acid is needed daily to improve the function of the adrenal glands. An exhausted gland can be linked to dry skin the Sjoegren's patient.
- Special supplements of raw adrenal tissue are available in health food stores and are of special importance for adrenal health.
- Daily use of raw seed oils is also very important. Example: Evening Primrose oil, Borage oil and Flax seed oil. Please refrigerate these oils after opening to avoid rancidity.
- Daily use of raw, unsalted and unsweetened nuts and seeds is equally helpful to provide the body with natural lubricants. Please, purchase only refrigerated nuts and seeds, preferably from a health food store. Any such products, displayed in open containers in supermarkets, are likely to be rancid and harmful to the patient. Please, refrigerate raw nuts and seeds and oils at all times.

# Systemic Sclerosis (Scleroderma) Localized Scleroderma General information

Systemic Sclerosis is subdivided into Diffuse Systemic Sclerosis (SS) and CREST

Diffuse Systemic Sclerosis

- Affects the circulatory system through changes in the blood vessels
- Causes inflammations which may involve internal organs and the skin
- Results in atrophy, wasting of otherwise normal tissue
- Causes the formation of abnormal amounts of collagen within an organ

CREST syndrome; also described as "limited". The word CREST is a combination of the first letter of each of these health conditions.

- Calcinosis—means abnormal accumulation of calcium in the skin
- Raynaud's phenomenon—a condition with affects the blood vessels

- Esophagus malfunction—especially that of the lower esophagus
- Sclerodactyly—means that abnormal tissue growth in fingers and toes has taken place
- Telangiectasis—means dilation of small blood vessels in the skin, often noticeable as small bumps close to the skin surface.

Both SS and CREST are considered to be a chronic autoimmune disease of connective tissues, which involves the overproduction of the body protein "collagen". Some as yet unknown mechanism triggers the extra growth of skin and tissue in organs, and this in turn affects normal function of these tissues.

# This is what medicine knows about Scleroderma

- Disease involves collagenous connective tissues
- As yet there is no one single known cause
- No current medical therapy can stop the disease.
- Some research focuses on the immune system, some on blood vessels and other research focuses on connective tissue itself
- Scleroderma is considered to belong to the family of rheumatic diseases
- Some researchers believe that SS is inherited
- The onset is slow and may take many years to develop
- Scleroderma is not contagious
- The majority of patients are middle aged, women, usually between 30 and 50
- Babies and young children are usually affected only by localized Scleroderma
- The disease occurs in all countries of the world.
- In the U.S. alone there are an estimated 300,000 or more cases. A recent internet publication however states that the two combined forms of Scleroderma are estimated to exceed 700,000

- Recent publications also imply that exposure to "Silica dust" may predispose a person to SS, while exposure to "vinyl chloride" can produce similar, but not true Scleroderma symptoms
- A cancer drug "Bleomycin" can also produce temporary Scleroderma-like symptoms

## Common symptoms of Systemic Sclerosis

- Overlapping symptoms of Sjoegren's syndrome (see "Sjoegren's section)
- Overlapping symptoms of Raynaud's Phenomenon (see section on Raynaud's)
- Overlapping symptoms of Systemic Lupus Erythematosus (see section on Lupus)
- Overlapping symptoms of Polymyositis (see section on Poly- and Dermatomyositis)
- There may be swelling of hands and feet
- There may be painful and stiff joints, making movement difficult
- Problems with the face
- Problems with the mouth, teeth and gums
- There may be weight loss
- General pain
- Extreme fatigue and weakness
- Trouble swallowing
- Blood vessel difficulties (see Raynaud's section)

## Systemic Sclerosis may affect only muscles, bones and skin, but not the internal organs, or…

- Affect many internal organs also, such as blood vessels, digestive organs, heart, lungs, kidneys and mucus membranes which line internal organs
- Can lead to heart problems. The disease can slow the heart down, cause chest pain, shortness of breath and can lead to heart failure
- Can lead to kidney problems, mental impairment, vision

problems, headaches and renal failure

- Can lead to pulmonary insufficiency, persistent coughing and shortness of breath
- Can cause damage to nerve endings, resulting in severe pain
- Can contribute to nutrient deficiencies in the thyroid, the adrenal glands and the liver. These organs become deficient in the very nutrients, which normally nourish cells of the epidermis, but no longer can do so because of the disease. Glands are needed for energy. Therefore a glandular malfunction results in the interruption of nutrients needed for skin circulation
- Can affect the face and hands before internal organs become involved.
- Patients, who also experience TMJ (temporal-mandibular joint) problems, should consult a dental specialist
- Can cause wide-spread, symmetrical, leathery, hardened or solidified skin areas. The appearance of the lesions verifies the presence of a systemic disease. This is later followed by atrophy (muscle wasting) and pigmentation (discoloration) of the skin.

## Summary

The majority of patients eventually will suffer involvement of the gastrointestinal tract, heart, lungs, kidneys, esophagus, and especially that of the skin and small blood vessels. A smaller number of patients will have problems with their stomach, intestines, with joints, tendons and muscles. Some suffer from high blood pressure.

## Common and typical CREST symptoms

- Calcinosis—accumulations of calcium found under the skin of fingers, knees, feet and arms. These sometimes erupt through the skin and can become infected.
- Raynaud's phenomenon—impaired circulation to the extremities, due to blood vessel spasms. Stress or outside

stimuli such as cold, heat and loud noises can contribute to this problem and cause spasms in the blood vessels of internal organs. Pain, tingling, burning sensations and numbness are characteristic symptoms. Raynaud's phenomenon is present in almost all Scleroderma patients.

- Esophagus problems—impairment of lower esophagus function, accompanied commonly by acid reflux episodes with resulting scarring of the mucus membranes. Many have been diagnosed with a hiatus hernia and simultaneous digestive upsets.
- Sclerodactyly—the skin of finger and toe digits becomes hard; fingers cannot flex. This often progresses to the fingers taking on a permanently flexed claw-like appearance.
- Telangiectasis—describes small raised red spots found especially on the fingers, palms, face and even the tongue. Some patients have reported these spots on the trunk and breasts as well. The spots are actually small blood vessels near the skin surface, and when viewed through a magnifying glass it becomes obvious that each spot consists of several tiny blood vessels.

Localized Scleroderma is divided into three forms:

- Morphea—this term is used for one or more plagues
- Generalized Morphea—a more serious form which may involve large skin areas, but does not affect other organs
- Linear Scleroderma

In Morphea characteristic hardened oval patches develop on the skin after an initial inflammation process. Morphea patches are light colored, ranging from white to yellow to ivory, surrounded by a purplish or violet border area. Morphea can affect almost all body surfaces, but is usually found on the trunk. This form of localized Scleroderma generally corrects itself in time. White, chalky looking small spots belong to a form of localized Scleroderma called "guttate Morphea" which does not occur as frequently as "Morphea".

Generalized Morphea is a much more serious form, but does not occur very often. This form of Scleroderma involves large skin areas. Fortunately it does not involve any other internal organs, nor does it have overlapping Raynaud's phenomenon symptoms.

Linear Scleroderma is characterized by thickened skin areas, which are usually found either on an arm or leg, but can also involve both sides and which can reach deep into the skin and affect underlying muscles and bones. Children with linear Scleroderma might have one strong leg, while the one affected by linear Scleroderma does not develop normally and remains weak. Such a band of abnormal, thickened skin might for instance reach from the hip down the leg to a foot, restricting movement. Such areas also suffer from loss of tissue. A deep cut-like crease is frequently found on the head or neck of Scleroderma patients. This very characteristic linear Scleroderma is called "en coup de saber" which translated means "strike by a sword".

Common symptoms of localized Scleroderma—Patients with facial and mouth involvement and those with temporal mandibular joint involvement may have the following symptoms

- "Fibrosis" areas in the tongue or palate
- Problems with the esophagus
- Thinning of the lips
- The tip of the nose can become thin, pointed and shiny
- Facial skin turns pale, becomes taut, inflexible and takes on a rigid mask-like appearance
- Muscles for the eye lids and those which normally make the cheeks flexible now lose their ability to move. This takes away a patient's ability to show emotions or feelings because the muscles needed to respond to emotions can no longer respond. The face eventually takes on a "frozen mask" look.

The patient goes to a medical physician. What happens next? Symptoms are usually reported to a general practitioner, and if the information provided by the patient is specific enough, he or she will be referred to a dermatologist and perhaps to a rheumatologist. As the problems worsen and organ involvement is obvious, all kinds of specialists get involved in the case and these will perform specific functions, depending on which organs are affected.

## Urologist—Kidney function

Many Scleroderma patients do not experience kidney problems, but those with severe hypertension must be closely monitored. Urine tests must be very specific to get correct results about possible kidney involvement.

## Cardiologist—Heart and circulatory function

Many patients have mild to severe problems, which are usually triggered by other internal organ malfunction. Lung function impairment for instance, can place great stress on the heart. Some patients also experience problems with fainting spells and frequent falls.

## Pulmonary experts—Lung function

Pleurisy episodes may occur, causing coughing and shortness of breath. Patients with esophageal problems have to guard against inhaling reflux matter into the lungs, a situation which could cause life threatening infection. If lung tissue is damaged, oxygen loss is a direct consequence.

## Gastroenterologist—For function of esophagus; hiatus hernia and intestinal problems

Scleroderma patients frequently suffer from malnutrition because of loss of function in the small intestines. This results in several problems. First, the patient does not get enough nutrition out of daily food intake, and secondly food is not digested correctly, remains in the intestines too long and grows an excess amount of harmful bacteria which can enter the blood stream and cause multiple health problems. The large intestine may lose its muscular function to move fecal matter towards the rectum. This can cause bloating and constipation.

## Specialist in liver diseases

While liver involvement fortunately is not common "viral biliary cirrhosis" does occur in some patients. This form of cirrhosis is now so common in Germany that specialty hospitals have been built for these patients. The eventual progression of viral cirrhosis leads to a liver transplant.

## Blood tests

Tests usually include a CBC and a test for the rheumatoid factor. A Westerngren sedimentation rate test, CPK muscle enzyme test and a test for antinuclear antibodies are other methods to test for Scleroderma.

## Nail cuticle test

The performance of small blood vessels is checked through a variety of tests, including the nail cuticle test

## X-ray studies

These are used to determine which internal organs are affected by the disease.

## Two major groups of drugs are used for the treatment of symptoms

- Drugs which aim at controlling or reducing fibrosis of organs and skin, such as D-penicillamine and Colchicine
- Specific measures focusing on organ and skin damages through Corticosteroids, anti-inflammatory drugs, drugs which dilate constricted blood vessels, and anti-

hypertensive drugs. These make up the major medical arsenal of weapons against Scleroderma.

Treatment measures include:

- Drugs which act as vasodilators
- Drugs which control blood pressure
- Lubricating crèmes for skin damage
- Antibiotics for infected areas
- Teaching patients how to use biofeedback for controlling impaired circulation
- Corticosteroids for arthritis-type pains and overlapping Myositis symptoms
- Special instructions to the patient to control reflux problems.
- Special instructions to patients with esophagus problems, difficulty swallowing and digesting foods (e.g. avoiding large meals, careful chewing and using plenty of drinking water)
- Dry mouth medicine and for bleeding gums und gum disease (please read Sjoegren's syndrome for information on natural medicines, such as CoenzymeQ10)
- The use of Captopril therapy for high blood pressure
- Physical therapy and exercise for body areas affected by localized Scleroderma
- Patients are instructed in correct exercise, how to avoid total fatigue plus other helpful information

Patients remaining under medical care only can contact these addresses for further information or guidance:

- Arthritis Foundation, 1330 West Peachtree Street, Atlanta, GA 30309. Ask for "Scleroderma brochure"
- Scleroderma Research Foundation, Pueblo Medical Commons, 2320 Bath Street, Suite 307, Santa Barbara, CA 93105
- Scleroderma Federation, Peabody Office Building, One Newbury Street, Peabody, MA 01960

# Discussion of Holistic Therapy Options
# Can alternative medicine help? General information

Holistic practitioners look at these facts:

- Skin function is impaired and this can have grave consequences for the Scleroderma patient
- The blood forming function of bone and lung tissue is disturbed and the body's response causes the blood to harden and to coagulate
- Nerve endings are injured; they malfunction and send severe pain signals to the autonomic nervous system (sympathetic and parasympathetic nerves) which then becomes involved in the disease process
- The thyroid glands, the adrenal glands and the liver are involved and can no longer supply those elements to the skin to keep it healthy and normal
- That when a shortage or absence of important hormones causes impaired glandular function, harmful germs (bacilli) are produced in the lymph vessels of the skin. As a result the skin layers "dermis" and "epidermis" become inflamed. The characteristic shiny skin seen in Scleroderma is caused by nerve damage to the skin.

- Glandular deficiencies affect lymph circulation, causing hardening of skin areas where lymph structures are destroyed. During the process of hardening the lymphatic vessels become irritated, inflamed and begin to create harmful germs. These germs destroy normal circulation and cause abnormal thickened malformations of tissue.
- During the advanced stages of the disease sweat glands malfunction, perspiration is impaired or stopped and the skin's normal breathing ability is destroyed. This results in acidosis, which makes the patient's body especially vulnerable to all kinds of infections.
- Advanced cases suffer from extreme oxygen deficiency, which puts every cell in the body under dangerous stress.

The reader is advised to thoroughly study all aspects of chapter III "Holistic Therapy Options". Knowing which specific nutrients can bring very specific help to ailing tissues is of immense value to the Scleroderma patient. ***Many specific and important nutrients and herbs are listed throughout this book. Some improve oxygen uptake, others naturally help the blood vessels to relax and dilate and by doing so improve blood circulation. Others bring important nutrients to the glands to ensure maximum output or to reverse an existing deficiency. ***While synthetic reproductions of Cortisone have been available for some time now and are used by medical physicians as anti-inflammatory medicine the body reacts to this "fake hormone" with great irritation. Prednisone, a form of Cortisone, is such a drug. While Prednisone can be tolerated somewhat for up to about ten days, the drug can produce severe side effects after that time span. The following serious side effects have occurred in patients:

- Changes in personality and swift mood changes
- Cataracts
- Glaucoma
- Elevated blood pressure
- Osteoporosis

- Bone necrosis (death of bone cells)
- Susceptibility to infections
- Severe fluid retention
- Ulcers
- Can worsen diabetes

Medical physicians caution against the use of Prednisone in patients over sixty years of age.

Methotrexate, a widely used immunosuppressive drug in all forms of connective tissue disease, has a terrible track record:

- Severe damage to lung tissue, liver and kidneys has been reported
- Severe bone marrow depression is possible
- Gastrointestinal bleeding can occur
- Mouth and throat ulcers have been reported after using Methotrexate.

Originally used for Psoriasis patients, this drug quickly gained a terrible reputation and, according to medical records, has caused deaths. Since many Scleroderma patients already suffer from liver involvement, the use of Methotrexate could be quite dangerous. ***The question is this: If holistic therapy can provide safe and natural alternatives, shouldn't the medical physician try these first and especially in non-crisis situations? And, shouldn't the patient have the right to be advised of safer options?

# Goals of holistic therapy for the Scleroderma patient

## Stimulate glandular action through

- Specific nutrient therapy
- Specific holistic therapy to those energy or nerve centers, which communicate with glands in the human body; for instance Acupuncture, Reflexology, Sacral-Cranial therapy, Chiropractic and other forms of energy healing.

## Thyroid gland

The thyroid gland is the body's temperature regulator. The feeling of extreme internal coldness in the blood vessels experienced by Scleroderma patients with overlapping Raynaud's phenomenon symptoms can in many cases be modified or corrected by taking tiny amounts of iodine, found in natural Kelp tablets or other sea vegetation extracts.

## Adrenal gland

The adrenal glands depend on optimum dosages of ascorbic acid for normal function. Pantothenic acid, also known as B5, is another essential nutrient for the function of these glands. The reader should know that the adrenal glands normally produce natural "Cortisone", a hormone substance which acts as an anti-inflammatory agent. Severe stress can deplete function of the glands and rob them of their ability to make this very important hormone. That is why orthodox medicine is using a synthetic form of the hormone, but sadly at a cost to the patient. So, when this hormone cannot be made naturally by the depleted adrenal gland the result is "inflammation". Please, read chapter V regarding the importance of ascorbic acid and why it is of such great importance to the human body.

## Promote assimilation through:

- A cleansing diet
- Correct digestion and assimilation problems through therapy from practitioners specializing in energy healing.

## Improve and correct peripheral blood and lymph circulation through:

- The use of specific nutrient therapy
- Any of the above mentioned energy therapy methods and/or consistent massage therapy
- Rubbing arms, hands, legs and feet daily with grain alcohol to stimulate lymph circulation
- Rubs with expeller pressed raw peanut oil (do not use hydrogenated oil). Starting at the sacrum rub down to the legs, also side to side, top and bottom. Rub Castor oil into hardened skin areas at least once daily; or apply Castor oil packs to the area, leave on for two hours, and remove for two hours; repeat this cycle often.

## Program to detoxify the blood stream

Patients can consult an herbalist, homeopathic or naturopathic physician for advice on specific herbal combinations to cleanse the blood of accumulated toxins. Water intake for proper cell irrigation is of great importance.

Improve oxygen uptake to help all affected tissue areas, such as the skin, lymph and blood. This can be done through:

- Use of natural vasodilators
- Correct exercise programs
- Yogi breathing techniques

Daily Castor oil packs (ref. Edgar Cayce readings)

- Saturate a piece of flannel with warmed Castor oil, place over entire abdomen starting at the diaphragm to just above pubic area
- Simultaneously place a Castor oil pack over the spine all the way down to the sacrum.
- Leave both packs on for two hours, resting during this time. Remove packs, sponge off with a sponge or clean rag soaked in "saturated bicarbonate of soda" solution.

Please, consult Edgar Cayce readings for more detailed information

Switch to a corrective alkaline diet

- Use plenty of green leaf vegetables, vegetable broths and vegetable soups prepared from organic materials.
- Avoid all fried foods
- Choose fish, poultry and lamb over any other meats

Daily Kelp supplements

- Kelp contains minute amounts of organic iodine plus other very important trace minerals. Using Kelp brings important nutrition to the thyroid glands and other body tissues to improve their function

## To build up strength

- Daily use natural red wine and rye crackers
- Daily use of egg yolk, beaten into glass of dark malt beer

## To normalize collagen production and to overcome sub-scurvy or acute scurvy blood levels

- Daily eat fresh, organic fruit high in vitamin C (ascorbic acid)
- Supplement with at least 3,000—5,000 mg of Ester C combined with Bioflavonoids. Increase to 10,000 daily
- Also use supplements containing cartilage. These are widely available in health food stores

## To prevent hardening of the skin

- Use high-grade vitamin E d-alpha tocopherol in 400 IU dosages two to three times daily with food. Please, read Dr. W. Shute's book "The complete and updated vitamin E book" for special cautions for patients with very high blood pressure and those with a history of rheumatic fever.
- Avoid using the synthetic form of vitamin E, identified by the letters dl following the letter E. These products will not bring the desired results. Rely on expert advice to choose the correct vitamin E

Stop inflammation of lymph vessels, blood vessels and the skin with natural anti-inflammatory substances (see chapter III for "natural anti-inflammatory substances").

## Strengthen affected organs

Kidneys, heart, lungs, joints and skin can be helped with specific nutrient and/or herbal therapy (see chapter III)

Soothe and protect irritated membranes of the esophagus:

- Use "Slippery Elm" lozenges. Let slowly dissolve in the mouth; then swallow.
- Use "Slippery Elm" herbal capsules for daily support.

- Drink plenty of quality water to hydrate all body tissues, including the mucus membranes lining the esophagus, stomach, intestines etc. Do not use distilled water which is void of all nutrients and not appropriate for drinking

## Other helpful information for the Scleroderma patient

- Dr. M.E. Barabash wrote in "Improvement of Scleroderma" Vestnik Dermatologii Venerology 32; 31, 1958 about his success with supplementation of 1,000 IU vitamin E daily, plus E oil applied directly to hardened areas.
- Another researcher wrote in an article about "Scleroderma in infants" that watery swellings, followed by infection, were very successfully treated with vitamin E.
- Dr. Wilfred Shute, M.D., in "Complete and updated vitamin E book", pg. 62, 85, 98, 217-219 quotes Cutis, 11/54, 1973 "Vitamin E successful in Scleroderma and Raynaud's Phenomenon with gangrene". "Vitamins E and A successfully used for Discoid Lupus Erythematosus".
- Vitamins E and A, both oil-soluble vitamins, can be used successfully for all connective tissue (collagen) diseases.

### Special notes about the importance of normal thyroid, parathyroid and adrenal gland function

Glandular function should be checked through appropriate medical tests but the results should also be evaluated by a nutritional counselor. Test results, which by medical standards still fall into the "normal range", yet either teeter on the extreme lower or upper end of that range, deserve a closer look. ***Adrenal gland malfunction can be a direct result of severe stress. Stress depletes the body of stored nutrients and quickly leads to nutrient deficiencies. The role of ascorbic acid and Pantothenic acid in normal adrenal gland function cannot be emphasized enough. Deficiencies in these nutrients certainly impact the Scleroderma patient. Hair analysis can also detect adrenal malfunction. ***Glandular malfunction caused by stress frequently results in "multiple allergies. Chronic yeast fungus infections, of which "Candida Albicans" is the most common, further challenge a Scleroderma patient's immune system and cause a condition of high toxicity and extreme sensitivity to many man-made substances such as vinyl products, chemical fumes, formaldehyde, artificial sweeteners and artificial food colors. *** Stress reduction is very important for the Scleroderma patient and other connective tissue disease patients. ***Thyroid under-activity is extremely common, because iodine and other essential thyroid nutrients are sadly lacking in today's diet. Other important trace elements, such as manganese and gold are also lacking. Both of these nutrients are important for healthy skin, joints, tendons, ligaments and membranes. ***A very common symptom of Scleroderma and other C.T.D. patients is the severe internal coldness they feel in their body tissues. This coldness, in the author's opinion and experience, is due to the shut-down of small and larger blood vessels due to the thyroid's inability to maintain normal body temperature. An iodine deficiency apparently throws this body heat regulator into a sudden and severe malfunction. Blood vessels react with a "slow-down" or a "temporarily complete shut-down". If this shut-down cannot be reversed, then eventually the affected tissue areas will die off. ***In some patients sugar binges will set off an episode of internal coldness. It is believed, that sugar binging upsets other glands which in turn affect the thyroid also.

Chronic yeast-fungal infections can cause frequent flare-ups of the disease, resulting in

- Pulmonary congestion
- Severe tissue pain
- Unbearable vaginal and groin itching
- Weeping and very smelly yeast lesions in the armpit and groin area
- Fevers, which often last weeks.

All body parts work together. If one malfunctions, all

others immediately try to adjust accordingly. It is therefore of benefit to the Scleroderma patient to experiment with various vitamins, mineral and trace element dosages until the correct (successful) dosage has been established and to switch to a healthy diet consisting of organic meats, fruit, vegetables and grains. ***Each patient has different nutritional needs. Therefore each C.T.D. patient, whether suffering from just Sjoegren's syndrome, Lupus or Scleroderma with overlapping symptoms from one or several of the others, has to find the right formula. It can be done, and it should be done.

Adrenal gland exhaustion stops or severely slows down the gland's production of the natural hormone Cortisone. This hormone acts as a natural anti-inflammatory substance. A patient with malfunctioning adrenal glands cannot handle stress at all or handles it very poorly. The reader is encouraged to carefully read chapter V, which deals with the extreme importance of supplementing with ascorbic acid and the role it plays in adrenal health.

# How certain nutrients and herbs can help the Scleroderma patient and other connective tissue disease patients

---

Vitamin E d-alpha—400 IU three to four times daily with meals. Please, read cautions for high blood pressure and rheumatic fever patients.

- Prevents gangrene
- Improves blood flow
- Thins blood naturally to prevent clotting
- Prevents hardening of tissue
- Acts as a natural vasodilator
- Counteracts certain liver and lung pathologies

Ginkgo Biloba—standard dosage two to three times daily

- Improves cerebral circulation and memory
- Improves peripheral circulation
- Acts as a natural vasodilator

Superoxide Dismutase (SOD)—follow instructions

- Prevents gangrene
- Improves blood flow

- Acts as a natural vasodilator

Dimethylglycine (DMG)—follow instructions

- Prevents gangrene
- Improves peripheral circulation
- Strengthens immune system
- Prevents ulceration
- Acts as a natural vasodilator

Ascorbic acid—minimum 5,000 mg in divided dosages

- Detoxifies blood
- Detoxifies liver
- Supports kidney function
- Stimulates lymph circulation
- Prevents hardening of tissue

CoenzymeQ10—four 100 mg capsules daily

- Cellular nutrient
- Counteracts any chronic disease process
- Reduces high blood pressure
- Supports the heart
- Supports lungs
- Supports kidneys and other structures

Manganese (trace mineral)—50 mg daily for at least 3 months; then reduce to 15 mg

- Strengthens tendon tissue
- Of special help in Osgood Schlotter disease

Cayenne

- Acts as a natural vasodilator
- Improves circulation

Ascorbic acid plus Pantothenic Acid (B5)

- Special support for adrenal glands
- To help patient to handle stress

Kelp—contains iodine and other trace elements

- Important support for thyroid glands

## Other helpful therapy for the Scleroderma patient

### For localized pain

- Arnica ointment or crème
- Arnica sublingual tablets
- "Blue Stuff"
- "Kool Comfort" by DeeCee Laboratories
- Reflexology therapy
- Acupressure therapy
- Acupuncture therapy
- Other energy healing therapies
- Mind over Matter exercises to control pain

### For Internal pain

- MSM
- Glucosamine sulphate
- Magnesium Citrate
- Many different natural anti-arthritis formulas are available in all health food stores
- Arnica
- Mind over Matter exercises to control pain

### Other helpful suggestions

- Colonic irrigations or liver flushes to remove toxins from system. Limit to 3 months intervals
- Natural yeast-killing medication
- Use of lactobacillus and other strains plus Lysine to rebuild beneficial intestinal flora and gain control over chronic yeast-fungal problems

# Systemic Lupus Erythematosus (SLE) Discoid (cutaneous) Lupus Erythematosus (DLE) Drug induced Lupus and Neonatal Lupus Lupus is an auto-immune disease

## Systemic Lupus Erythematosus SLE

- Lupus occurs worldwide
- An estimated 75 persons per million in America become ill with the disease each year
- Outbreaks are especially prominent during spring and summer sun exposure (UV rays)
- Patient's immune system malfunctions and attacks its own healthy tissue
- SLE is a chronic, inflammatory disease of connective tissue, usually for the rest of the patient's life.
- All patients have constant flare-ups and remissions
- At times there may be no sign of the disease
- Inflammatory means: pain, heat, redness and swelling
- Patients can live a full life in some cases, but many SLE medications produce severe side effects.
- According to medical information SLE cannot be cured but symptoms can be controlled with potent medication.

SLE affects multiple organs, such as:

- Joints
- Central nervous system
- Heart
- Kidneys
- Liver
- Lungs
- Brain
- Blood, blood vessels and skin

Discoid or cutaneous Lupus Erythematosus (DLE)

- SLE is a benign skin disorder, which normally runs its course during a 10-20 year period
- An estimated 1 million individuals suffer from this form of Lupus
- It is less dangerous than SLE, but a disfiguring skin disease, which produces small, soft, yellowish lumps on the skin
- There can be raised, red, scaling lesions with raised edges and plugged follicles. These lesions can affect the face and ears, scalp, neck, arms and other body parts and can cause atrophy and scars
- Hair can become brittle
- There can be hair loss
- DLE may be chronic
- DLE produces a characteristic butterfly shaped rash on cheeks and nose
- DLE may be limited to the skin and not be associated with diseases of other body systems
- Some DLE cases are part of SLE
- Patients must wear protective clothing against sunlight, avoid prolonged exposure to the sun, avoid fluorescent lights and should remain indoors between 10 AM—4 PM.
- Very recent reports state that a solution prepared from one teaspoon ascorbic acid and two tablespoons water may be applied to the skin, allowed to air dry and that this

solution appears to protect better than any sun screen
- Silver crème can also be used or sun protection

Drug induced Lupus
- Lupus-type symptoms can develop from taking certain medications.
- Once the drug is discontinued symptoms usually disappear within a reasonable amount of time.

## Causes of systemic Lupus Erythematosus (SLE)

At this time no single cause for Lupus has been identified by orthodox medicine. Some researchers present the following information:
- SLE is considered to be an auto-immune disease
- SLE is considered to be an abnormal body reaction to the patient's own body tissues; evidently caused by a faulty auto-immune system which produces ANA (anti-bodies) from antigen anti-body complexes. These anti-bodies poison cells and interfere with normal immunity. In Lupus anti-bodies may form without the presence of bacteria
- A genetic predisposition to the disease exists and certain factors can cause the disease to develop, such as mental or physical stress, strep or viral infections, immunizations or pregnancy. Some families evidently produce several generations with this genetic predisposition. More than one case can occur within a family unit. Yet, other researchers say, there is no evidence that a parent passes it on to a child. They believe that a virus triggers the genetic tendency to develop Lupus.
- The disease can be triggered by certain drugs. Listed are "Procainamide", "Hydralazine", anti-convulsant drugs, sulfa drugs, penicillin and oral contraceptives.
- Medications for high blood pressure, heart disease, seizures and psychological problems can cause many of the symptoms and may result in abnormal blood tests. These symptoms usually disappear upon discontinuance of the medication. (Reader, please note that the author

stated in an earlier chapter the relationship between large doses of penicillin and the onset of auto-immune disease)

- Some studies suggest that some patients develop SLE after a long and especially stressful time. Stress depletes the body of ascorbic acid and contributes to sub-scurvy symptoms. This leads to exhaustion of the adrenal glands
- People on oral contraceptives or receiving hormone replacement therapy, some during a pregnancy, and others just during a menstrual cycle; have reported that this is how their SLE started.

A major cause in the author's opinion is the discovery and subsequent gross overuse of penicillin and other antibiotics, which in years past were prescribed for even the slightest sniffle. This caused an epidemic of chronic yeast-fungal infections. These chronic infections are due to massive organ infiltration by harmful yeast fungi resulting in extreme tissue toxicity, multiple allergies and connective tissue changes. The situation is further complicated by chronic and substantial ascorbic acid deficiencies. The entire body is under attack all the time causing, for instance frequent ear infections in babies and children or constant bladder infections in women. And usually these infections are once again treated with more antibiotics. ***It appears that so far nobody has investigated "systemic fungal infections" as a possible contributing cause for Lupus. And because fungal infections are a serious health threat to Lupus patients and other patients suffering from auto-immune diseases, the author encourages the medical community to thoroughly test each individual C.T.D. patient for evidence of all types of chronic or active fungal infections. ***Anyone interested in more information may request the results of a private study of eleven patients, all diagnosed by medical physicians with one or more auto-immune diseases. The author found that all of the study participants had repeated and extensive antibiotic therapy since childhood and many viral and fungal infections throughout their lives.

## Who is most prone to develop Lupus?

- Majority of patients are female
- First signs usually occur during child bearing years
- Lupus can also occur in children and older people
- Dark skinned people are more frequently affected (only one of 400 white women, but one in 250 black women are affected)
- The disease usually strikes between the age of thirteen (puberty for most) and the age of forty-five

## SLE—First symptoms as the illness begins:

- Fatigue
- Weakness
- Fevers; usually low grade
- There might be weight loss
- Sometimes loss of hair
- Some patients develop mouth sores
- Some cases begin with arthritis, swelling and pain in fingers and joints

## As the illness progresses, the following symptoms can develop:

- Skin rashes on the arms, neck and face
- A characteristic facial erythema (rash) in the form of a butterfly involves cheeks and the nose
- Photosensitivity develops. Patients become very sensitive to UV rays. Their rashes grow worse after exposure to sunlight
- Fingers become very sensitive to cold, turn a blue color. This symptom also occurs with Raynaud's phenomenon, an illness which can occur simultaneously with Lupus.
- Some patients develop "Vitiligo", a loss of pigment. Depigmented areas on the arms or other body areas also may turn a bluish color from exposure to cold

- Oral ulcers develop
- Ulcers appear in the nasopharyngeal area
- Ulcers of mucus membranes are common in Lupus
- Lymph node enlargement, diffuse or local, but not painful
- Parotid gland swelling, very painful; pain sometimes radiates into the front of the neck and can also affect the ears and chewing ability and contribute to "Trigeminal Neuralgia"
- Abdominal pain
- Loss of appetite
- Nausea
- Vomiting
- Diarrhea or constipation
- Irregular menses
- Amenorrhea, a problem which occurs during flare-ups
- Joint pain in the hands, wrists, elbows, knees and ankles. Deformities are not common
- Feeling of inner tightness and stiffness in joints and/or muscles, when patient wakes up. This symptom might occur right along with joint pains
- Alopecia
- DLE symptoms may also be present (butterfly rash)
- Raynaud's phenomenon symptoms may be present
- General pain
- General muscle aches
- Frequent or constant fever, usually low grade from one to four degrees above normal
- Spiking fevers
- Chills which may last just a few seconds or last for several hours
- Hair loss
- Painful breathing
- Swollen glands
- Severe skin rashes
- Severe fatigue

Advanced cases may present these additional symptoms:

- Increased tendency towards frequent infections
- Nose bleeds
- Anemia. These patients experience weakness, are short of breath and pale
- Some patients develop blood clots
- Many patients experience an inflammation of the lining of some body part; heart, lungs, stomach, interior abdominal wall and interior rib cage can be affected. All can result in severe shortness of breath and pain
- Kidney problems are common. In the early stages of Lupus kidney problems may not be obvious, but later swelling of the legs indicates, that protein is present in the urine. Please, see very special section on "holistic therapy for the kidneys".
- Vasculitis
- Infarctive lesions (including kidneys)
- Leg ulcers
- Digital gangrene
- Symptoms of Raynaud's phenomenon are seen in roughly 20% of SLE patients

## The following organs can suffer serious damage

### Heart and Lungs—symptoms

- Cardiopulmonary abnormalities in 50% of patients
- Pleurisy, an inflammation of the pleura
- Pericarditis; an inflammation of the heart sac
- Dyspnea; shortness of breath
- Myocarditis; inflammation of the muscular walls of the heart
- Endocarditis; inflammation of the lining membrane of the heart
- Tachycardia; excessively rapid heart beat
- Parenchymal infiltrator; essential tissue of an organ
- Pneumonia

## Kidneys—symptoms

- Renal abnormalities are common in Lupus and may lead to kidney failure
- Hematuria
- Proteinuria
- Urine sediment
- Cellular casts
- Nephritis; inflammation of the kidneys
- Renal thrombosis
- Renal infarction

## Other urinary system symptoms

- Repeated ureter tube infections
- Repeated bladder infections
- Repeated urethra infections
- All symptoms are due to SLE patients' susceptibility to infections

## Central nervous system involvement can result in mental or neurological problems:

- Emotional instability
- Psychotic episodes
- Organic brain syndrome
- Irritability
- Moderate to severe and deep depression
- Trouble focusing, concentrating
- Mood changes, often rapid
- Medical physicians report certain abnormal behavior in some patients, which they believe could be caused by the illness itself or could be the patient's reaction to the illness. Disfiguring scars or having to deal with the prospect of death can be too much of a mental burden for some patients.
- Very few patients develop more serious mental problems, but they do occur occasionally

- Convulsive-type seizures similar to epilepsy can occur, but are rare and usually go away

## Blood abnormalities

- Anemia
- Low white blood cell count
- Decreased platelet count
- Elevated ESR
- Serum electrophoresis, hypergamma-globulnemia

## What causes repeated flare-ups?

- Recurring chronic systemic fungal infections are suspected to cause a flare-up of Lupus symptoms
- Sun exposure can be a trigger. UV rays can cause flare-ups but can also cause the very first attack
- Other infections in the body can trigger a flare-up
- Fatigue
- Childbirth can bring on a new attack
- Certain drugs cause flare-ups
- Some patients experience flare-ups after dental anesthesia
- Certain chemicals are suspected, e.g. working with computers, scanner and printers
- Unidentified viral infections
- Menstruation cycle can cause flare ups
- Birth control pill can cause flare-ups
- Hormone replacement therapy can be a trigger
- Some patients have flare-ups after being exposed to formaldehyde fumes in particle board and other materials containing this chemical and various glues used in modern lumber products

Getting a clear diagnosis is difficult. Misdiagnosis is common because the symptoms of Lupus mimic those of many other diseases. This is especially true for the beginning of the disease. Patients feel misunderstood and often are labeled "neurotic" by both physicians and family alike because of the multitude of different symptoms nobody seems to be able to explain. ***A correct diagnosis can take several years, especially for older patients. The disease usually develops and evolves slowly over a period of many years. Many of the symptoms come and go, making it difficult for both patient and physician to see a clear pattern. ***An accurate diagnosis in milder cases is very difficult, because there is not one single test that provides a clear diagnosis. Very thorough questioning by the physician during an examination can provide some clues. ***According to a recent internet publication about Lupus, physicians use a list of eleven criteria. It appears from this article, that the patient must meet at least four of those to be assured of a correct diagnosis. Seven of the criteria involve symptoms; the other four are lab tests (see below).

- Chest x-rays—can provide information about possible lung or heart involvement
- ANA test—the blood is tested for antibodies. 95% SLE patients have a positive ANA. On the other hand, if a patient has many of the symptoms listed but has a negative ANA, then a diagnosis of Lupus is quite unlikely. But, physicians caution that a positive ANA alone is not enough proof of Lupus, since a positive ANA is also found in rheumatoid arthritis. Sjoegren's syndrome, Scleroderma (both connective tissue diseases), Mononucleosis, Malaria, sub-acute bacterial Endocarditis (infection processes) and both auto immune thyroid and liver diseases can also produce a positive ANA. A positive ANA by itself, the doctors say, does not positively identify an illness, because it can be found to be positive in individuals who have no illness.

Since the disease evolves slowly and mimics many other health problems during its development, it is quite difficult for a general practitioner to diagnose Lupus. A well informed patient, who suspects he/she has the disease, can request a referral to a rheumatologist or immunologist to receive the benefit of more detailed testing. ***As stated, about 95% of Lupus patients have a positive ANA. Only a very small percentage has a negative ANA, but in many of these patients other antibodies are found in the blood, such as antiphospholipid antibodies, anti-Ro and anti-SSA. ***An ANA can also be influenced by steroids, cytotoxic medications or uremia medication.

## Anti-DNA

- Most specific for SLE, is rarely positive in other conditions.

## LE cell tests

- Are positive in most active SLE cases

## EKG

- Can show conduction defect

## CBC

- Provides information about white blood cells, red blood cells or platelet counts and nutritional status

## Kidney tests

- Urine analysis
- Collect urine for examination
- Possible kidney biopsy (which might show the extent of renal involvement)
- Liver function test

Often patients are sent to a psychiatrist, because multiple complaints without outward evidence are misinterpreted by physicians as "neurotic" complaints. These patients are not taken seriously; the physician may simply ignore the long list of complaints. Some patients spend agonizing, frustrating long years, trying to convince their doctors that they are really sick.

The presence of the following symptoms will enable the physician to make a definite diagnosis:

- Mouth sores
- Abnormal cells in the urine
- Arthritis type symptoms
- Butterfly rash
- Sensitivity to the sun
- Seizures
- Psychotic episodes
- Low white blood cell count
- Low platelets
- Hemolytic anemia
- Presence of specific anti-body found
- Profuse protein urea (3.5 g/day)

Additionally urine studies (WBC's and RBC"s, urine casts sediment tests and significant protein loss C3 and C4 indicate active disease. There may be excessive cellular casts in the urine.

# Discoid Lupus Erythematosus (DLE) Common symptoms

### Rashes—Butterfly rash

- A rash with either flat or raised lesions, which can cover both cheeks and the nose. Sometimes it can appear as a bright red, sometimes just a pinkish color. Its outline resembles that of a butterfly.

### Rashes—Discoid rash

- Usually develops on skin areas that have been exposed to too much sunlight, such as the front and back of the neck, lower arms and hands. This rash is disk-like, either coin or oval shaped. Sores, developing from this rash become scaly and red. They frequently leave a scar. The skin surrounding the remaining scars undergoes color changes and may either turn or dark in color. These lesions can also be found on the scalp and the face and can take on the characteristic butterfly appearance.

## Rashes—Sub-acute cutaneous lesions

- A third type of Lupus rash has been identified as "sub-acute cutaneous lesions". These lesions are red, round, very sensitive to light and actually worsen when exposed to UV light. This rash can appear on large body areas, but does not leave scars behind. Patients experience fever, a general ill feeling, muscle and joint discomfort and other symptoms.

## Diagnostic procedures for Discoid Lupus Erythematosus

- DLE requires a dermatologist for an accurate diagnosis.
- Skin biopsies may be necessary to reach a definite diagnosis, since there are so many different rashes involved.

## How Lupus can complicate other diseases

- Patients with osteoarthritis may experience more joint damage and pain
- Lupus can cause patients to have heart attacks and strokes earlier in life
- Lupus is a severe and often unpredictable disease. It causes depression in many patients, because of the complexity of their disease

## Some people develop additional health problems from taking Lupus medication for many years, such as:

- Osteoporosis
- Cataracts
- Glaucoma
- Ulcers
- Infections
- Fragile skin

  All of the above can be made worse by steroids.

## Common medical treatment for Discoid Lupus Erythematosus (DLE)

- Usually some ointment or Corticosteroid crème, which is applied to the lesions. If unsuccessful, steroid injections may be used
- In extensive lesions the patient frequently receives oral Corticosteroid medication, and the physician might prescribe Plaquenil (hydroxychloroquine).
- Patient will be advised to use strong sun screens and avoid direct sunlight. Direct sun exposure can activate new rash episodes.
- There are US companies, which specialize in protective clothing for such patients

## Medication for DLE is prescribed according to need and severity of illness

- Aspirin or other anti-inflammatory drugs
- Non-steroid anti-inflammatory drugs, such as "Clinoril", "Feldene" and others are mentioned in the American Arthritis Foundation folder. Both aspirin and NSAID's can damage the liver and kidneys
- Anti-malaria drug "Plaquenil", similar to"Quinine" is commonly prescribed. This drug, according to the pamphlet, is helpful with DLE, but also for some of the SLE symptoms, such as joint pains, fever and inflammation of lung lining. However a caution is issued: long-term use can cause blurring eye sight and blind spots.
- Corticosteroid drugs are used for severe Lupus cases. This very potent medication can greatly reduce the pain of inflammation. Side effects are weight gain, bruising, depression, mood swings, the typical moon face, insomnia, high blood pressure, edema and swollen lips, complicating existing diabetes, increasing risk of infection and making osteoporosis worse.
- Prednisone is used to control inflammation, but can cause

spacyness, trouble remembering and in some patients weight gain. Cases of bleeding stomach have occurred in connection with long-term use of steroids.

- Immunosuppressive drugs –These drugs are used to treat active, severe auto-immune disease and usually are combined with steroid treatment. Serious side effects have been observed. Known drugs are "Imuran", "Cytoxan", "Chlorambucil", "Methotrexate" and "Cyclosporine". Patients taking these medications must be monitored closely by their medical physicians. Immunosuppressive drugs are used especially for advanced kidney problems.
- Kidney failure—may require daily kidney dialysis or even a kidney transplant to save the patient's life.
- Treatment for infections may be necessary.

## Further guidelines for Lupus patients

- Exposure to sunlight or fluorescent lights can cause Lupus rashes to get worse.
- Sun exposure can cause a sudden flare-up. When this happens, the immediate reaction can be joint pains, fever, inflammation of the heart, lungs, kidneys or the nervous system. Doctors advise Lupus patients to avoid direct sunlight and stay indoors between 10 AM and 4 PM. Lupus patients living in the warm southern states can purchase special sun-protective clothing.

Women with Lupus during their child bearing years may experience difficulties with both pregnancy and contraceptives. Medical advice for these women is as follows:

- Use the safest contraceptives, such as a diaphragm with contraceptive jelly.
- Oral contraceptives are o.k. in some cases based on individual evaluation.
- Miscarriages are common
- Women may experience their first Lupus sign with their first pregnancy.

Women, who already have Lupus and then become

pregnant, may experience a more severe form of the disease. This again seems to indicate that the hormonal balance has a great effect on such a patient. Current information states that doctors advise pregnant women to have a check-up for antibodies, because a transfer from mother to fetus through the placenta can take place. The effect on the baby would be a rash, low blood count and possibly enlarged liver. Usually the symptoms go away by the 6th month. ***Patients are also advised to restrict protein intake to prevent kidney malfunction and edema; to rest when the illness flares up and to seek a balance between rest and activity.

### To summarize the four drug categories:

- Steroids, including Prednisone
- Non steroidal anti-inflammatory drugs
- Anti-malarial medications
- Chemotherapy

### SLE patients should notify their physician at once if any of the following symptoms occur:

- Seizures or convulsions
- A very stiff neck and accompanying headache
- A fever higher than usual
- Unusual bruises on the body
- Vomiting
- Blood in the stool
- Feeling of being extremely irritated or aggressive
- Feeling confused; can't get thoughts together
- Any kind of chest pain
- Kidneys do not produce urine
- Pain in kidney region

### What are the patient's survival chances from a medical point of view?

Depending on whether a patient has a mild, moderately

severe or very severe case, doctors maintain that the majority of patients can lead a reasonably normal life and live out a normal life span. Severe cases can eventually become fatal. However, medications used for the treatment of Lupus can have grave side effects and perhaps contribute to a premature death. ***Recent clinical studies focus on a genetic linkage as well as the evaluation of DHEA (male hormone) and the role it could play in patients with Lupus. There are many other studies done world-wide which hopefully will give the public more satisfactory answers about this disease. Lupus patients, interested in medical research, should take advantage of the tremendous wealth of information available on the internet, especially in regard to support organizations, research centers and other important sources of information.

## Drug induced Lupus (DIL)

Some common drugs can cause Lupus-type symptoms

### Hypertension drugs

- Taken for long periods of time may lead to drug-induced Lupus, a mild form of the disease

A recent internet publication listed the following drugs which may also lead to drug-induced Lupus

- Procainamide (Procan) and (Prenestyl)—used for heart rhythm abnormalities
- Hydralazine (Apresoline) and (Apresazide)—used for high blood pressure
- Isoniazid (INH)—used for heart rhythm abnormalities
- Penytoin (Dilantin)—used for convulse disorders

While the author has provided the reader with in-depth information about medical views and current treatment of connective tissue diseases, a major goal of this book however, is to provide the patient with alternative therapy options in non-crisis situations and offer some hope for a better future by educating the public about safe and natural solutions. Usually only medical advice is available to patients. But with the information presented patients could make important decisions to use medical treatment only, combine natural therapy with medical treatment or rely totally on alternative medicine only. for life extension and especially quality of life. ***The following section on holistic therapy for the Lupus patient hopefully will lead the way to a healthier life.

# Discussion of Holistic Therapy Options
# Can holistic therapy help the Lupus patient?

---

## Holistic guidelines for mild cases of Lupus

- Rest is of great importance. Patients need a minimum of eight hours of sleep
- Daily walks, preferably several short ones rather than one long tiring walk. Such a walk should begin slowly, stretching first followed by deliberate swinging of the arms to stimulate the pulmonary-cardiac system and to stimulate brain function
- Cross crawl exercises are equally important for normal brain function. Instructions on how to: When walking the left leg and right arm move forward, then right leg and left arm etc. When walking is not possible, this exercise can be done standing in place or even sitting in a chair
- Food intake should focus on a high fruit, high vegetable and whole grain diet and the use of raw nuts and seeds for their wholesome fats and essential fatty acids which help to avoid platelet aggregation and are of importance for the prevention of strokes. All fresh shelled nuts and seeds should be kept in a tightly closed container and

refrigerated at all times to avoid rancidity, because rancid oils cause destruction of vitamin E. Nut and seed oils and olive oil used for cooking should be cold-pressed (expeller-pressed) and always refrigerated for the same reason. Please, avoid all hydrogenated oils, margarines or any product prepared from such fats. They are a risk factor in blood clot formation. These fats called "trans fats" cause platelet aggregation which can lead to sludgy and clotting blood.

- Red meats should be used very sparingly, and if used must be cooked slowly and thoroughly. Red meats can place a great burden on the kidneys which are under great stress in about half of all Lupus patients.
- Fish, poultry, rabbit meat and organic eggs are better animal protein choices than red meat.
- Nuts and seeds offer the most valuable form of protein
- Eggs (organic) can be used moderately. These are especially well tolerated beaten into a favorite soup or vegetable stew.
- Protein intake must be monitored to avoid kidney overload.
- Butter can be used sparingly; one to two tablespoons per day.
- Drinking lots of water is absolutely essential for kidney irrigation. Please, do not use distilled water for drinking or cooking. Also avoid osmosis filtered water.
- Along with a supportive diet the use of a complete mineral and vitamin supplement is still of immense value, since the Lupus patient has problems obtaining all essential nutrients from regular food intake.
- Additional use of ascorbic acid, CoenzymeQ10 and Ginkgo Biloba is strongly recommended by holistic counselors.
- Daily use of yogurt (health food store variety only) to support a healthy intestinal flora

## Holistic guidelines for moderately to severely ill Lupus patients

- All of the holistic guidelines for mild cases of Lupus are equally important to the moderately or severely ill patient. In addition this information is being offered:
- All known allergens must be avoided to reduce stress to the immune system. This includes food, chemicals, yeast, mold, mildew or any other substance which causes a strong reaction in a patient. Severe cases may have to use steroids or immunosuppressive medications from time to time. Patients must be aware, that it is dangerous to suddenly withdraw from steroid medication. When experiencing side effects from steroids such as hair loss and weight gain, many patients become discouraged and abruptly discontinue their medication. It is dangerous to do so without an evaluation by the attending medical physician.
- While holistic therapy encourages the use of a high vegetable and fruit diet, Lupus patients should stay away from "Alfalfa sprouts". They contain "Canavain" a natural toxin which incorporates itself into protein in place of the amino acid Arginine.
- Helpful and effective teas for Lupus are: Echinacea, Goldenseal, Pau d'Arco and Red Clover.
- Effective for arthritis-like symptoms in Lupus are: Yucca and Alfalfa seed tea.
- Many severely ill SLE patients suffer from kidney impairment. (Please read the special holistic section in this book devoted entirely to kidney therapy).
- Water intake is of the utmost importance for all human beings, but in time of great physical stress becomes a life extending force. To repeat an earlier statement: "Distilled water is not acceptable". Quality drinking water from a certified source or home-filtered water is the only option. Commercially sold drinking water filtered by osmosis, should also be avoided because it is low in minerals.
- Patients with active yeast-fungal infections must adhere

to a strict yeast diet, which may restrict even fruit and fruit juices because of their sugar content. Please, consult chapter III for natural anti-fungal therapy options. ***Chapter III "Holistic Therapy Options" provides lists of

- Natural, safe anti-inflammatory substances
- Natural, safe anti-pain therapy
- Natural, safe antibiotic substances
- Natural, safe vasodilators
- Natural, safe antioxidants
- Natural, safe tranquilizers
- Safe, natural substances for neurological problems
- Safe, natural substances for the brain and mind
- Safe, natural substances for kidney and bladder problems
- Safe, natural substances for cardiovascular and pulmonary problems.

These natural substances can be added to orthodox treatment or substituted for many of the dangerous medicines except for crisis situations. When combining medical prescriptions with herbs it is necessary to check with the pharmacist first. ***In the author's opinion, holistic therapy gives patient hope for a better life. While this approach may work too slowly for many suffering folks, it can and will reward the patient with better quality of life in the end. ***The list of natural and safe substances can be used for symptoms suffered by Lupus patients and those of other connective tissue diseases. And each patient has to make a decision whether to stay with current orthodox medical treatment as the only form of treatment, to combine medical and holistic therapy or to use holistic therapy only. ***A patient with advanced SLE symptoms, experiencing great pain and other symptoms should remain with allopathic medicine, provided a clear diagnosis was given and the patient was informed of all possible severe side effects of medications used. If these medications can offer a patient some relief, then why not use them? On the other hand it must be understood, that these very drugs can cause additional serious health problems and at the same time trick the patient's body into feeling better, while the disease continues to progress. It will be a difficult choice to make.

The human body is capable of healing itself and most disease processes can be reversed with some help. These are the building blocks:

- Correct diet
- 2 quarts of quality water daily to irrigate all cells and help detoxification
- Appropriate exercise, especially daily walking
- Correct breathing techniques for optimum oxygenation (e.g. Yogi breathing)
- Daily use of positive affirmations to reinforce the healing process
- Use of specific nutrients to repair and strengthen weak tissues
- Use of biofeedback to further enhance the healing process
- Use of natural therapy to re-establish normal energy flow (chi energy). Reflexology, acupuncture, acupressure, Reiki and many other forms of energy healing are very effective.

# Suggested nutrient supplementation program for SLE and DLE Lupus patients

- Ascorbic acid (vitamin C) in Ester form plus Bioflavonoids—1,500 mg three times daily with meals; needed for normalizing collagen and to strengthen immune system
- Vitamin E d-alpha tocopherol—400 IU three times daily with meals (do not substitute synthetic vitamin E which can be identified by the letters dl). Vitamin E d-alpha is a natural antioxidant, oxygenates the blood and is needed to keep the blood at the correct viscosity and to prevent blood clots. Patients with very high blood pressure and a history of rheumatic fever must read cautions (see chapter III) Vitamin E is very effective in preventing vasospasms, which occur in Lupus and Raynaud's phenomenon.
- A multi-mineral supplement, which must contain all gross and trace minerals (example: Mezotrace). In addition minerals in colloidal liquid form are of great value, since they are assimilated immediately.
- Amino acids: L-Cystine—important for normal skin cell growth and white blood cell activity; Tyrosine—important

for skin cell growth, melanin and white blood cell activity; L-Cysteine—assists in cellular protection and preservation; L-Methionine—assists in cellular protection and preservation. A complete amino acid supplement, which includes proteolytic enzymes and HCL to reduce allergy reactions would be most helpful and the best solution, rather than trying to take individual amino acids.

- B6 (pyridoxine)—works with magnesium to prevent seizure activity; also helps to prevent tendonitis, bursitis and carpal tunnel symptoms
- B-complex 100 mg, three times daily with meals to provide energy; improves brain function and helps prevent neuralgia and neuritis. If a patient suffers outright neuralgia pain (e.g. Trigeminal Neuralgia) B12 taken in liquid form taken under the tongue is of great help.
- Vitamin A in emulsified form only—50,000 IU daily—a powerful antioxidant
- Zinc picolinate in chelated form—30 mg three times daily with meals; protects immune system and is very important for continued good eye health.
- Superoxide Dismutase (SOD)—known as a powerful antioxidant.
- Sulfur—used for weepy skin conditions. Eggs and onions are good natural sources of sulfur.
- CoenzymeQ10—important cell nutrient and used in Europe and Japan to treat and prevent congestive heart failure or to prevent heart disease. Q10 is of great importance to the Lupus patient; Normal maintenance dosage is 30 mg per day; for acute illness physicians recommend 400 mg per day in divided dosages. Best taken as a spray under the tongue for immediate assimilation.
- Ginkgo Biloba—to maintain or improve cerebral circulation, improve memory and maintain a good mental attitude. Ginkgo Biloba is also of great value in restoring normal circulation to legs and feet.
- Acidophilus and other bacilli strains for recovery from

yeast-fungal infections and to restore normal intestinal flora. Combined with Lysine it is of great value when yeast infections become weeping sores (often seen under women's breasts, under abdominal fatty folds, in the groin or arm pits). Colloidal silver or Aloe Vera can be used topically to treat the lesions. . Raw garlic or in tablet form is of great help in restoring normal intestinal flora.

## Other helpful tips using holistic therapy

- Daily use of colloidal silver as a natural antibiotic
- Daily use of flax seed oil to prevent blood clots and platelet aggregation
- Flax seed oil, Borage oil, Evening Primrose oil and fish liver oils all supply Omega 3 and Omega 6. These substances are helpful in decreasing skin inflammations and are important skin nutrients. Essential fatty acids found in these oils are especially important to prevent blood clotting or thick blood. This is especially important for the patient with kidney impairment, because renal thrombosis or renal infarct can occur in advanced Lupus patients.
- Daily use of a homeopathic tissue salt supplement which contains all twelve tissue salts for normal body function. It must not be confused with a mineral supplement. Tissue salts were discovered to be the very components all body cells are made of. Disease, according to Dr. Schuessler, results from inherited weaknesses and subsequent vulnerability to certain disease processes. The tissue salts strengthen and normalize imperfect tissues by bringing the cells slowly but surely back to optimum function. A supplement containing all twelve salts or individual salts for specific conditions are available at all health food stores.

# The importance of using the right fats

The fats listed below are of great value to all patients suffering from connective tissue disease because they nourish the skin from within and help diminish the painful rashes of Lupus. They also prevent platelet aggregation (blood clots). But only raw unsalted and unsweetened nuts and seeds provide this help because the nutrients have not been destroyed through heat or other processing.

- Sunflower seeds; pumpkin seeds; squash seeds; safflower seeds. Raw seeds must be refrigerated in closed container to avoid rancidity
- Almonds; walnuts; hazelnuts; filberts; pistachio; cashews. and Brazil nuts. If possible nuts should be purchased in the shell and refrigerated. When purchasing shelled nuts they should be kept in a closed container and refrigerated to avoid rancidity.
- Seed and nut oils: raw, expeller pressed oils should be used only. Refrigerate after opening. These oils can be used daily as follows: one tablespoon added to salads, soups, stews and cooked vegetables.

Please, avoid all products containing hydrogenated oils. They are dangerous to your health!

# Special Kidney Section Holistic therapy for kidney and urinary tract problems

## Part I. General information

The kidneys are expected to process about 500 gallons of blood during a 24 hour period. Blood circulates continuously through the entire body When it reaches the kidneys, water and proteins are purified, given back to the system, while unusable materials, excess fluids and excess nutrients are being dumped into a couple of tubes, which connect the kidneys with the bladder. These tubes are called "ureter tubes". The ureter tubes take urine to the bladder. When the bladder is full, a signal goes to the little tube called "urethra" which first signals to the person that it is time to go to the bathroom; then the sphincter of the urethra opens and allows the urine with waste materials to be expelled. Anything that interferes with kidney or bladder function, can have disastrous consequences for the patient. ***What can and often does go wrong with kidneys and bladder in connective tissue disease? Gravel (tiny kidney stones) and kidney stones (clumped together gravel) can cause great pain in the ureter tubes and bladder. Gravel or sand usually passes through without difficulty. However, when this gravel aggregates (clumps together) in either the kidney or the bladder, then the patient experiences severe pain. If kidney stones leave the kidney, but get stuck in one of the ureter tubes, urine loaded with waste materials cannot get through. Kidney or bladder stones have sharp edges and can damage the soft lining of the tubes and cause absolutely agonizing pain. But when blockages occur and waste cannot be eliminated the body quickly becomes very toxic. The patient is in great danger. ***Medical treatment includes pain medication to relax the patient and allow the stone to pass through on its own; surgical removal or pushing the stone back into the kidney and using ultrasound to break up the stone into small particles, which then can pass through. Stones can also form in the bladder and cause damage there.

## Cystitis occurs in the bladder

The mucus membranes lining the inside of the bladder sac can become inflamed. These membranes then begin to defend themselves by making extra mucus in an attempt to fight off harmful germs and various salts. Patients with this problem observe very cloudy urine and experience a deep ache in the lower abdomen with pain extending into the small of the back. Urine release may become very painful, slow down and sometimes stops altogether. No doubt that medical help is needed here. In women this condition is usually caused by bacteria accidentally being wiped from the rectum into the nearby opening of the urethra because the two openings are so close that fecal bacteria can enter very easily.

## Urethritis

Urethritis is an inflammation which occurs in the little tube "urethra".

## Ureteritis

Ureteritis is an inflammation which occurs in one or both ureter tubes; the tubes which connect the kidneys to the bladder.

## Nephritis

Nephritis is an inflammation or infection of the kidneys.

## Renal vein thrombosis

Clotting of the renal vein causes engorgement of the vein and can result in renal infarction. If both kidneys are involved and a sudden thrombosis causes malfunction in both, the patient's life is in great danger. If only one kidney is involved or if a thrombosis develops gradually then partial kidney function may continue. The most obvious symptoms are severe lumbar pain, pain in the epigastric area and pain under the ribs. Immediate medical care is of great importance, whether such symptoms are relatively mild or severe.

## Renal infarction

A renal infarction occurs when kidney blood vessels become occluded. Emergency medical care is needed. Symptoms:

- Severe upper abdominal pain
- A gnawing flank pain or tenderness in the flanks
- Rib pain
- Gastric upsets
- Fever

# Part II

## Holistic therapy options for kidney, bladder and other urinary tract problems

It is very important that all herbs are purchased from reputable sources only. Patients must pay careful attention to dosages and other instructions to determine, if an herb can be used for short periods of time only and other important safety guidelines. Please, consult a naturopathic physician, homeopath or experienced herbalist for the correct use of herbal remedies. Do not rely on inexperienced persons for advice! Patients are advised not to self-treat without specific instruction by a qualified professional. If pain develops or urine production slows down or stops during herbal treatment, it must be considered a crisis situation which demands immediate action. In mild cases herbal teas can be used to relieve the condition. However, more severe cases must be evaluated and monitored by qualified health professionals.

### "Compound tea" combination from the Heung San area in China can be used for the following conditions:

- Helps to dissolve and expel small kidney stones
- Helps to dissolve and expel gravel
- Relieves kidney inflammation
- Relieves bladder inflammation; relieves kidney blockages caused by albumine
- Relieves some ureter tube and urethra conditions

  For bladder irritations, gravel, sand, stones and cystitis:
- Fo-Ti-Tieng root tea. Tea also tones up bladder
- Parsley Piert
- Buchu tea
- Shepherd's purse; sage; marshmallow leaves; peach leaves—use a mixture of these
- Parsley tea

- Flaxseed
- Fenugreek
- Watermelon seed (black seeds) tea. For women only
- Corn silk tea

### Chronic cystitis, a bladder irritation caused by phospatic and uric acid gravel:

- Corn silk tea

### Bladder drip:

- Corn silk tea

### To increase flow of urine

- Corn silk tea

### Frequent urination, especially at night is usually caused by Candida albicans infection:

- Buchu tea

### Urine has strong odor, is scant with heavy sediment. This is a sign of kidney inflammation:

- Strong corn silk tea

### Bladder infection:

- Watermelon seed tea (best is black-seeded). Not recommended for males

### Scalding urine

- Juniper berry mixture (Short-term use only)
- Shepherd's purse
- Corn silk tea

### Kidney infection, kidney inflammation:

- Juniper berry tincture, tea or oil ( Short-term use only)
- Sage (purifies kidneys)
- Equal parts of sage and peppermint leaves

## Nephritis, a kidney inflammation

- Parsley tea

## Kidney infection, urinary tube infection, bladder infection:

- Fresh or bottled cranberry juice; 6 ounces three times daily. Children 4 ounces three times daily

## Kidney stones

- Parsley tea

## Ureteritis affecting ureter tubes and urethra lining

- Parsley tea
- Juniper berries; buchu; clivers; marshmallow leaves; sage; uva ursi; parsley piert. Crush 1 oz. each into fine powder. Please, ask professional about daily dosage.
- Corn silk tea
- Shepherd's purse

## Fluid retention

- ½ ounce couch grass and ½ oz. knot grass

## Antiseptic for ureter tubes, bladder and urethra:

- Uva ursi tea
- Sage

## To restore mucosa of inflamed irritated urinary tubes:

- Marshmallow tea

## Mucus in urine, cloudy urine:

- Shepherd's purse
- Mixture of shepherd's purse, sage, marshmallow leaves and peach leaves

# Vasculitis in Lupus Erythematosus General information

Medical research divides Vasculitis in the Lupus patient into two categories:

A) A reaction by the immune system

In this case the immune system reacts to "antigens", certain substances which trigger an allergic reaction. The body detects the antigens and begins to produce "antibodies" (proteins). These antibodies attach themselves to the antigens and form what is known as "immune complexes". How does the body destroy antigens? By either relying on white blood cells or other body substances.

B) An actual infection of the blood vessel walls

Apparently this is not very common. When it occurs, some immune complexes somehow cannot perform their job and gradually infiltrate blood vessels. Their presence irritates the blood vessel walls and causes inflammation. It has been found that in Vasculitis white blood cells which normally destroy harmful invaders, can also accidentally destroy blood vessel tissues. ***The substances involved in creating these immune complexes in Lupus patients are not always clearly identified. One antigen recently discovered in an immune complex was named “anti-neutrophil cytoplasm antibody”. A recent internet discussion disclosed that this antigen can cause Vasculitis in some Lupus patients.

## Common symptoms of Vasculitis

- Fatigue
- Feeling of general unwellness
- There may be joint and muscle pain
- Patient might have a poor appetite and weight loss might occur without trying to lose weight
- Petechia is common; small red or purplish colored spots, most frequently found on the legs but also on the trunk of the body. Magnified one can recognize blood seepage
- Purpura; a larger version of Petechia, usually between ¼ and ½ inch in size
- Areas of what looks like bruises
- There can be very itchy rashes
- Some patients have small black spots at the tips of their fingers or in the tissue surrounding the nails. These are small infarcts
- Joints can swell, become warm and painful
- In cases involving the brain severe headaches, seizures as well as a stroke can occur. Such a patient may also show sudden behavior problems
- Neurological symptoms may involve impaired sensations to the extremities, such as numbness, tingling or weakness. Weak grip of the hands and weakness in the ankles is common
- Slow blood flow to the intestines can cause cramping, bloating and pain. If impaired blood flow to the intestines causes gangrene, surgery is an absolute must. These cases also show blood in the stool
- Usually the heart, lungs or kidneys are not affected by Vasculitis. Recent research reports that even Lupus patients with nephritis are not affected by Vasculitis.
- The retina of the eye can be affected. Blurring vision or partial vision loss can occur.

Medical treatment varies, depending on symptoms and severity and will not be discussed in detail. However, the usual treatment consists of corticosteroids or pain medication. The reader is encouraged to read the following information about "holistic therapy options".

# Discussion of holistic therapy options for the Lupus patient

## Can alternative methods work?

The action of vitamin E as a natural vasodilator has been discussed in detail throughout this book. In the author's opinion any nutrients, herbal substances or other natural substances which are capable of keeping blood vessels from constricting are worth considering as a natural treatment. ***Dr. Wilfred Shute, M.D. Cardiologist, Canada, the famous vitamin E researcher, published his important findings regarding the beneficial effect of vitamin E on all types of skin and blood vessel conditions. The reader is encouraged to carefully study his book "The complete and updated vitamin E book" for detailed information. ***Important research published by Dr. S. Ayres describes the successful treatment of skin conditions with vitamin E in Raynaud's phenomenon, gangrene, Scleroderma, Calcinosis cutis and several types of cutaneous Vasculitis and Lupus. ***Ulcerated, denuded areas can be treated with vitamin E d-alpha tocopherol supplements with dosages ranging from 800 IU to 1600 IU daily. Patients should also apply a mixture of 50% vitamin E oil and 50%

Flaxseed oil to the skin. Or the patient can use 100% strength vitamin E oil on a small skin patch to test for possible reactions, because some patients are allergic to the full-strength oil. If no reaction occurs, then full strength vitamin E oil can and should be applied at least twice daily to all affected wounds. ***Vitamin E research in dermatology has resulted in many beneficial applications. Patients affected with Vasculitis are encouraged to try supplementing and external application with vitamin E for repair of connective tissue and growth of new by-pass blood vessels as described in Dr. Shute's book. Existing scars can be softened and sometimes completely eliminated with vitamin E oil. New scars can be prevented with the same treatment. ***Patients with symptoms of Vasculitis, Raynaud's phenomenon, SLE or Scleroderma benefit in many ways from vitamin E supplementation, because vitamin E oxygenates the blood stream and improves the body's ability to heal itself in many situations. ***An open wound can be treated several times daily with Aloe Vera gel. When the gel has dried vitamin E oil is applied. The wound then is covered loosely with sterile gauze. ***Chapter III will provide additional information about vitamin E and its many functions in the human body.

# Primary and Secondary Raynaud's phenomenon and Raynaud's disease

## Primary Raynaud's phenomenon

The cause is not known. It affects both hands and both feet but has no connection to other connective tissue diseases. Primary Raynaud's phenomenon is less harmful than Secondary Raynaud's.

## Secondary Raynaud's phenomenon (serious form)

Occurs with other diseases

## Raynaud's disease

Is considered to be one of several arteriospastic diseases

## Terms used in talking about Raynaud's phenomenon and Raynaud's disease

- Blood vessels; arteries (large); arterioles (smaller) and capillaries (tiny) Capillaries are the connection between arteries and veins. Distributed throughout the body, they are in charge of bringing oxygen and nutrients to body tissues

- Connective tissue diseases affect joints, blood vessels, skin, tendons, ligaments, periosteum (membrane overlying bones), muscles, cartilage and internal organs
- Antibodies; made by the immune system to fight and neutralize bacteria, viri and other harmful invaders. Abnormal antibodies are called anti-nuclear antibodies. These are found in patients with connective tissue problems. They attack the center of a healthy cell. They attack the body instead of defending it
- Vasospasm; this describes a sudden narrowing of blood vessels and is caused by muscles contracting resulting in insufficient blood flow. In Raynaud's the smooth muscle in blood vessels contracts (spasms) reducing or shutting off blood flow. This in turn causes the skin of the affected area to turn a white color, then blue. When blood flow resumes, the skin turns very red for a while.
- Ulcers and lesions; a change in skin tissues. The skin becomes abnormal because of insufficient blood supply.
- Gangrene; gangrene in Raynaud's phenomenon describes the process of tissue dying due to blood flow stoppage. In some patients toe or finger digits develop gangrene and have to be amputated

## What is Raynaud's phenomenon?

- It is usually called a disorder of those blood vessels which supply the skin. Responding to certain outside stimuli, these blood vessels will suddenly contract, stopping or limiting blood flow. The medical term is "vasospasm".
- Patient experiences little or no pain
- Affected area tingles, feels numb, and some report a feeling as if ice water is running through their blood vessels.

Secondary Raynaud's phenomenon has been linked to:

- Smoking, which also causes Buerger's disease
- Drugs
- Sjoegren's syndrome
- Systemic Lupus Erythematosus (SLE)
- Scleroderma
- Rheumatoid arthritis
- Arteriosclerosis
- Pulmonary hypertension
- Interference to nerves supplying the muscles
- Certain injuries, such as frost bite and surgery

Secondary Raynaud's phenomenon occurs simultaneously with other connective tissue diseases, such as:

- Sjoegren's syndrome
- Systemic Lupus Erythematosus (SLE)
- Scleroderma
- Rheumatoid arthritis (RA)
- Polymyositis
- Dermatomyositis

## Is there a cure?

- Medical science offers no cure but claims that it can control the disease. However, if gangrene cannot be stopped by medicine, then the disease is not being controlled; alternative medicine on the other hand offers some relief
- Usually attacks do not occur all the time and rarely leave lasting damage to body tissues. The exceptions are those patients, who have frequent and quite severe episodes.
- Biofeedback can be effective in stopping a vasospasm

## How does it affect the patient?

- Wherever blood flow stops, the skin will turn white. Next, the skin will turn blue because the stagnant blood remains in the blood vessels

- The most common symptoms are pain, a feeling of numbness and extreme cold. Some patients describe this feeling as "ice water running through their veins".
- There may also be a deep aching and a tingling feeling
- When blood flow returns, the skin can turn beet red or even purple
- The return of blood is often described as a "sudden rush of warmth, as if "liquid heat" is running through vessels. Some people describe it as "throbbing, pulsating".
- If blood flow does not return gangrene can occur which may require amputation of affected digits

Secondary Raynaud's phenomenon produces more serious symptoms:

- There may be problems with swallowing. The muscle of the esophagus may be weak and affect normal swallowing of food and drink
- The ankles may feel very weak and will not hold up the person. The feet have a tendency to collapse outward, putting great strain on the legs. In the author's opinion this weakness is caused by a severe ascorbic acid deficiency which weakens all connective tissue. The tissues cannot and will not perform in a normal fashion, until the deficiency is corrected
- The wrists may feel very weak. Trying to twist open a jar may cause agonizing pain, because the tendons, muscles and ligaments of the wrist cannot do their job. At that moment they are "imperfect tissues", again caused by a gross ascorbic acid deficiency.
- Along with pain a patient might feel that the muscles are glued together and that they cannot be stretched. When this occurs in the rib cage, it can make breathing very difficult and gives the patient a feeling as if a steel band is tightened around the chest. Evidently the periosteum (the membrane overlying the bones) is affected by the disease

and cannot function in a normal fashion. There may be severe pain when this occurs.

- When it occurs in the legs, or in the back of the neck or skull, it might feel like a taut internal band, so tight that no amount of stretching can bring relief.
- Some patients experience a sudden release of copious amounts o saliva accompanied by an unusual sour or acid taste
- Some patients describe an internal tightening of the inner abdominal wall, making it extremely difficult to stand upright. Patient wants to lean over from the waist to relieve some of the pain.

## Without medical treatment or holistic therapy the following situation can develop:

- In some patients blood circulation cannot be restarted. Usually this occurs in the extremities. The affected tissue then turns black, looks like tar and dies. This condition is called "dry gangrene". Many patients will lose the last digit of their fingers or toes; or areas of "dry gangrene" appear on their feet.
- Ulceration also can be a big problem when destruction of tissue develops. These ulcers are usually difficult to treat and may take a long time to heal when orthodox medical treatment is used.
- Holistic (alternative) medicine offers help. Please, study all holistic entries carefully.

## Medical versus holistic treatment goals

- Medical treatment goals are directed towards preventing tissue damage. This is not always successful. If the illness progresses to gangrene, surgery may be needed to remove the affected dead tissue. Medical treatment may include: Calcium channel blocker "Nifedipine" to open blood vessels and "Phenoxybenzamine" to block adrenaline effect on the blood vessels.

- Holistic treatment goals focus on the repair of damaged tissues and the formation of new cells and most of all, to avoid the development of gangrene. Certain key nutrients can be of immense help to the patient.

## How does medical science diagnose Primary Raynaud's phenomenon?

- The physician looks for signs of tissue deterioration, such as ulceration, gangrene or pitting scars.
- The cuticle-nail fold test is negative
- The ANA test is negative
- The ESR test is negative
- The patient reports having blood vessels spasms for at least two years. These vasospasms are described as blanching (skin turns white), cyanosis (skin turns blue) and flushing (skin turns beet red).

## How does medical science diagnose Secondary Raynaud's phenomenon?

- Capillaroscopy: oil is placed on the nail cuticle. If there is a change in the capillaries. Test is positive
- ANA test: this test determines if the body is making antinuclear antibodies. Test is positive
- ESR test: this test determines if inflammation is present and how fast red cells settle out of the blood. An elevated ESR means inflammation is present and the test is positive.
- The patient has repeating episodes of blood vessel spasms. . Test is positive
- There are signs of skin damage, such as ulceration, pitting scars, gangrene in fingers, toes and other parts of the hands and feet

## What can a patient do to avoid or minimize vasospasms?

- Smoking and caffeine have a "constricting" effect on blood vessels and can cause vasospasms
- By not operating any tool or instrument with strong vibrations such as a riding or push mower, tractor, chain saw, weed eater and brush cutter, electric drill, electrical massage unit, musical instrument with strong vibrations (such as the deep powerful tones of an organ or electrical guitar), or traveling in an automobile or jet plane.
- A chronic Raynaud's phenomenon patient may be very sensitive to loud music and loud noises of any kind. Listening to hours of high-pitched whining coming from a neighbor's mower or being exposed to the throbbing powerful speakers of a teen's car can actually cause a vasospasm.
- Since exposure to cold can bring on attacks, it is important that the body, hands, feet and head are kept warm and protected against cold air and cross drafts. Cold air of air conditioners can also cause vasospasms. Gloves, hats, scarves and warm socks should be worn during cool and cold days.
- Wearing wide, comfortable shoes is helpful. Sandals with lots of toe room are ideal. Any tight and constricting shoe should be avoided, as well as socks with toe seams to avoid irritation to the foot tissues.
- It makes sense not to go barefoot except on smooth and flat surfaces. However, most Raynaud's patients experience discomfort, when their feet contact a cool or cold floor.
- Natural fibers, such as cotton, wool and flannel are preferable to synthetic materials
- If needed, several layers of clothing may be helpful, just as layering of bedding may be needed to keep the patient comfortable.
- The extreme inner coldness experienced by Raynaud's patients usually doesn't respond to local heat application.

However, if the entire body surrounding the blood vessels can be warmed, it eventually will have a beneficial effect on constricted blood vessels (see holistic treatment options)

- Patients with dry skin will find help in the holistic treatment section
- By avoiding all tightly fitting garments, because they may interfere with circulation
- During an acute attack the finger tips might be so sensitive to heat or cold that the patient can actually sense a temperature difference between a flannel shirt and the button. The button will feel cold and send a pain signal to the patient's finger
- By avoiding playing all string instruments during an attack, since the pressure on the finger tips can cause great discomfort and possible harm
- While much is written about the effect of cold on the Raynaud's patient, many experience severe pain when fingers make contact with hot water. So, it is not just a question of avoiding cold items. The nerve endings evidently are extremely sensitive to heat as well and over-react
- Many physicians advise their patients to move to a warm climate. The holistic point of view is however to direct efforts towards normalizing tissue function rather than having to move. Besides, it gets cold in the desert too and sun exposure must be limited anyway
- Playing piano, accordion, organ and any instrument requiring prolonged finger contact can bring on new vasospasms
- Stress control is of the utmost importance, because severe stress can trigger an attack. Relaxation techniques and biofeedback can be used to reduce stress. Visualization exercises are also helpful
- Many physicians prescribe "calcium channel blockers" to relax smooth muscle tissue and to dilate capillaries. "Alpha blockers" work by counteracting the action of

norepinephrine, a hormonal substance which constricts blood vessels

- "Nitroglycerine" has also been prescribed, which is applied to finger digits to prevent gangrene and to heal ulcerations. But not all patients are helped. Usually it is the patient with the more severe Secondary Raynaud's phenomenon who does not respond well.
- Daily exercise is absolutely essential

## Besides coffee and smoking, certain medications must also be avoided:

- The American Arthritis Foundation suggests that headache medicines which act as vaso-constrictors must be avoided. (Examples: "Ergomar" "Ergostat", "Medihaler" and "Ergotamine").
- "Alpha-Beta Blockers" used for angina, high blood pressure and migraine headaches, such as "Inerdal LA", "Corgard", "Lopressor", "Trandate", "Normodyne", "Sectral" and "Blocardren" are to be avoided
- Adrenergic stimulators used for colds and respiratory problems must be avoided, such as cold tablets, "Triaminic" and "Naldecon".
- Balch & Balch in "Nutrition Healing" warn against the use of birth control pills
- Cancer chemo-therapy
- Recent research identified workers who are exposed to "vinyl chloride" to develop a Scleroderma-type illness, which can be part of Raynaud's phenomenon. This information was obtained from an internet chat room of Raynaud's patients, who discussed medications they were taking and additionally from an internet publication addressing the very same problem.

Please, carefully study the following pages which discuss the holistic therapy approach to Raynaud's phenomenon and disease and the use of safe and natural substances in non-crisis situations and for prevention.

# Discussion of Holistic Therapy Options for Raynaud's phenomenon and disease

## Vitamin E d-alpha—how it works

- Anti-oxidant
- Increases oxygen to tissue
- Increases blood flow
- Prevents and treats existing gangrene
- Dissolves fresh blood clots
- Prevents blood clots
- Prevents and treats sclerosis of the legs
- Dissolves existing fresh clots in the heart, lungs and arteries

Suggested dosage: 400 IU with meals: three times daily for two weeks; then 400 IU four times daily.

Caution: hypertensive patients and those with a history of rheumatic heart disease must limit their dosage to a maximum of 40 IU daily. Dosages are based on research by W. Shute, M.D. and Evan Shute, M.D., Canada

Evening Primrose oil—how it works

- Prevents platelet aggregation (follow instructions on container)

### Hawthorn berry extract—how it works

- Increases blood flow
- Improves oxygenation
- Prevents spasms in Angina patients
- Follow instructions on container

### CoenzymeQ10—how it works

- Antioxidant
- Greatly increases cell life
- Increases stamina
- Very important for prevention and treatment of heart disease
- Very effective for treatment and prevention of congestive heart failure
- Increases oxygenation of blood
- Increases blood flow

Suggested dosage: 30 mg daily for maintenance; 30 mg four times daily for acute or critical illness: 100 mg four times daily for chronic and advanced illness until improvement is seen.

### Acidophilus—how it works

- Important for anyone using antibiotics to restore intestinal flora and to fight existing yeast infections

### D.M.G. (Dimethylglycine)—how it works

- Prevents gangrene (Russian medical research)
- Prevents strokes, especially T.I.A.'s (Russian medical research)
- Antioxidant (Russian and US research)
- Increases oxygenation (Russian research)

- Prevents/treats leg ulcers (Russian research)
- Strengthens both branches of the immune system. (Russian research)

D.M.G. was formerly known as "pangamic acid" or B15

## Kelp—how it works

- Strengthens thyroid ; contains iodine and other important trace elements
- Maintains normal blood clotting activity because it contains vitamin K
- Helps regulate internal thermostat (heat and cold)
- Helps to normalize metabolism
- Kelp is effective for internal coldness during vasospasms

## Alfalfa—how it works

- Alfalfa also contains vitamin K and helps maintain normal blood clotting
- Has powerful detoxifying effect on entire system

## S.O.D. (Superoxide Dismutase)—how it works

- Powerful antioxidant
- Increases peripheral circulation and is of special importance to the Raynaud's patient.
- Derived from green vegetables and sprouted grains and seeds. Available in tablet form.

## Ginkgo Biloba—how it works

- Increases peripheral circulation, Aids mental processes and, like S.O.D. is of special importance to the Raynaud's patient and other C.T.D. patients

## Cayenne—how it works

- By eliminating mucus forming foods and adding Cayenne to daily food an immediate improvement in circulation can be observed
- Increases fat metabolism
- Hot Chili peppers increase metabolism by causing sweat

and a more effective way of burning calories (e.g. 45 calories of a 700 calories meal)

## Ascorbic acid (vitamin C)—how it works

- Extremely important for collagen production
- Normalizes damaged blood vessels
- Extremely important for repair of inferior or damaged muscle, tendon and ligament tissues (chronic ascorbic acid deficiency has been linked to rheumatic diseases, such as "Lupus", "Scleroderma" and other connective tissue diseases).
- Helps the body to detoxify many harmful substances. Vitamin C neutralizes many toxic metals
- Mega-doses have a definite therapeutic effect on patients suffering from connective tissues disease (collagen diseases). Dr. Linus Pauling suggests a daily minimum of 10,000 mg in divided dosages to ensure constant availability to the cells.

# Raynaud's disease
# General information

- It is considered to be one of several primary arteriospastic disorders
- Affects women more often than men, usually between puberty and age 40
- Constricts and causes spasms to the blood vessels in the fingers, toes, tip of the nose and other body areas
- Can cause "dry gangrene" in an affected body part
- Characterized by episodes of vasospasms in the small peripheral arteries and arterioles
- These episodes can be brought on by exposure to cold. For instance, touching ice or picking up a cooled item from the refrigerator can cause a vasospasm
- Some patients experience vasospasms touching very warm or hot substances
- Raynaud's disease occurs bilaterally; usually affects the hands, less often the feet.
- Very common in smokers. Can occur even years after a person has quit smoking
- Medical physicians consider Raynaud's disease a benign condition, which means they do not consider it necessary

to provide specific treatment and that they do not expect it to develop into a serious condition

- Raynaud's disease can best be described as "poor blood flow to fingers, toes, nose tip, ears and sometimes internal organs"
- If no other symptoms than those mentioned are present, the condition is classified medically as "Raynaud's disease" in contrast to the much more serious Raynaud's phenomenon.
- A vasospasm can last from just a few minutes to several hours

Holistic treatment options for Raynaud's phenomenon are appropriate for Raynaud's disease also.

# Polymyositis—Dermatomyositis Inclusion Myositis—Juvenile Myositis

(All are "Inflammatory Myopathies")

## General information

- Both Polymyositis and Dermatomyositis are considered to be systemic auto-immune diseases.
- Cells which are capable of causing inflammation actually surround normal healthy muscle fibers, then penetrate the fibers and finally destroy them outright. This results in weakness of the affected muscle areas. Cells attacking healthy body tissue are also found in other connective tissue diseases such as Systemic Lupus Erythematosus (SLE), Sjoegren's syndrome and Scleroderma.
- The onset may occur quite suddenly or can take months, sometimes even years
- The earliest signs are that the patient finds it difficult to get up quickly; it may be difficult to raise the arms to comb one's hair or to dress; patient has difficulty walking up stairs and is quickly fatigued when having to stand long or

walk a distance
- There can be difficulties with breathing and/or swallowing
- Mainly there is weakness and inflammation of muscles
- Inflammation causes impaired function and subsequent weakness of affected tissues
- Myositis affects connective tissues in muscles, cartilage, tendons, ligaments, internal organs and blood vessels.

## Polymyositis

### General information

Polymyositis is considered to be a systemic auto-immune connective tissue disease. The cause of the illness is unknown according to medical research. Medical testing includes:
- A thorough physical examination
- Looking for skin lesions (red-purplish erythema on elbows, knees and finger joints)
- Muscle weakness in either the lower or upper extremities and the trunk
- Phantom pains (sudden shooting pains) in muscles with accompanying fever
- Specific blood tests to verify a diagnosis
- Muscle biopsy
- Electromyography testing
- Test for elevated serum creatinine
- Test for elevated serum aldolase
- Test for elevated CPK

### Common symptoms

- In contrast to Dermatomyositis Polymyositis does not produce a rash
- Average patient age is 50 to 70 years
- Twice as many women as men have this disease
- Disease sometimes develops very quickly, but can take years in some patients

- The muscles closest to the trunk are first affected; other muscles can be affected later on
- Difficulty breathing
- Difficulty swallowing
- Problems with constipation or colitis
- Problems with the abdomen
- Death in adults can occur from progressive muscle weakness and respiratory failure

## Medical treatment

- Corticosteroid medication, usually for a period of up to 6 weeks
- Upon improvement the medication is reduced. Maintenance is achieved with Prednisone for the rest of the patient's life
- Patient who do not respond to Corticosteroids may be given immunosuppressive medication instead

Please, study holistic therapy options for all connective tissue diseases.

# Dermatomyositis
# Dermatomyositis is an auto-immune disease
# General information

Common symptoms

- A characteristic patchy purplish-red, dusky rash
- Most often seen on the knuckles (finger joints), knees, elbows, the bridge of the nose, on the upper chest and the back
- Hardened, calcified bumps can be felt under the skin. These bumps are frequently the first sign of a developing muscle weakness
- Less than half of patients have trouble swallowing
- Muscles closest to the trunk are affected
- Some patients experience breathing problems because of muscle weakness
- Children with Dermatomyositis usually have more problems with pain than adults

Medical treatment

- High dosage Prednisone (immunosuppressant) is commonly used
- Other immunosupressants are Methotrexate and

Azatioprine. Both have severe side effects.

- Some physicians use immunoglobulin given by I.V. with some success

# Inclusion Myositis General information

Disease is similar to Polymyositis and characterized by muscle weakness

- According to recent information a muscle biopsy is the only accurate test to differentiate between Polymyositis and Inclusion Myositis
- This illness usually develops very gradually after the age of 50
- Physicians believe that there is evidence that some patients may have inherited the problem
- There is no known treatment according to the most recent publications
- Physicians usually prescribe physical therapy only

# Juvenile Myositis (Juvenile Idiopathic Inflammatory Myopathy) General information

- There are characteristic rashes which usually appear before weakness in the muscles closest to the trunk develops
- Muscle weakness develops slowly
- Patients commonly have trouble swallowing
- Hoarseness or raspy voice are a common symptom
- There can be stomach pain
- There can be arthritis-type pain

Medical treatment

Corticosteroids are used for both Inclusion and Juvenile Myositis.

# Discussion of Holistic Therapy Options for the Myositis patient

Alternative health practitioners view Myositis as a condition which is secondary to another disease, such as Systemic Lupus Erythematosus (SLE) or Raynaud's phenomenon. In order to achieve symptom relief for Myositis the primary cause must be eliminated first. Only then can beneficial results for the treatment of this problem be expected. Holistic therapy focuses on the following treatment goals:

- To enhance circulation by providing appropriate nutrient formulas, specific nutrients and/or herbs
- To overcome inflammation by using appropriate specific nutrients and/or herbs
- To help relieve pain with specific herbal formulas, individual herbs or specific nutrients in specific dosages
- To strengthen the immune system through specific nutrients or herbs
- To address muscle weakness and neurological problems

## Circulation

- The reader is encouraged to look up the chapter "Holistic Treatment Options" and find "natural vasodilators" and other information on how to improve circulation, such as shown for Raynaud's phenomenon

## Inflammation

- Please, consult the chapter "Holistic Treatment Options" and locate the entries for "natural anti-inflammatory substances". MSM (Methylsulfonylmethane) for instance, is well known for its natural anti-inflammatory but also for its pain relieving effects. MSM's pain relieving action equals or surpasses that of Tylenol.

## Pain relief

- Again, the reader is encouraged to study the chapter "Holistic Treatment Options". This large chapter lists many natural substances, which can help to relieve pain. Important listings include MSM, but also Glucosamine Sulphate which has been researched by many well-known physicians. G. Douglas Andersen, D.C. for instance, wrote a wonderful article in "MPI Dynamic Chiropractic" 10/21/94 issue. The article stated that Glucosamine sulphate relieves joint pain and inflammation, increases range of motion and is much more easily assimilated than other forms of Glucosamine. And, contrary to many non-steroidal anti-inflammatory medical drugs, Glucosamine Sulphate has no side effects. Arnica, a homeopathic pain reliever, taken orally, can also be of help.

## Rashes

- The rashes of Dermatomyositis have been treated successfully with an ointment made of crushed and pulverized CoenzymeQ10 mixed with just enough Olive oil to make a thin paste. Mixture is applied often. (Ref. Italian research).
- Vitamin E oil can also be applied directly to such rashes
- Aloe Vera Gel has been used with success
- Vitamin C crème (available from health food stores) is another valuable holistic option for treatment

## To strengthen the immune system

- The chapter "Holistic Treatment Options" contains many valuable entries.
- CoenzymeQ10 is a major cellular nutrient needed in all chronic disease processes to strengthen the immune system.
- D.M.G. (Dimethylglycine), researched by Russian scientists, helps both branches of the immune system and is important for both chronic and acutely ill patients.
- Both CoenzymeQ10 and D.M.G. are also of vital importance for patients with circulation problems, heart problems and/or for the prevention of minor and major strokes

Muscle weakness and neurological disturbances, such as muscle coordination problems and burning and tingling sensations can be addressed with holistic therapy

- Patients with muscle weakness should ask their physician to test for a possible B12 deficiency. The most accurate test is a urine methylmalonic acid analysis by gas chromatography and mass spectrometer. Muscle weakness, neuralgia pains and many kinds of neurological disturbances can be caused by a B12 deficiency.
- B12 is available in liquid form (taken under the tongue), B12 injections (available from both naturopathic and medical physicians) or in tablet or lozenge form; however, B12 in this form is not easily assimilated.
- Muscle weakness can also by caused by a locked sacrum or problems with cranial sutures. Therapists practicing cranial-sacral therapy are particularly suited for addressing this problem.

# Mixed Connective Tissue Disease

Patients who have been diagnosed with "mixed connective tissue disease" may have some, but not all Scleroderma symptoms; may have some but not all of the Lupus Erythematosus symptoms; have some but not all of either the Primary or Secondary Raynaud's phenomenon symptoms; have some but not all of the Polymyositis symptoms. Because of the overlapping symptoms, "mixed connective tissue disease" cannot be classified as a single disease.

The reader with multiple symptoms is encouraged to read this book carefully and apply whatever holistic therapy fits specific categories of distress.

## Fibromyalgia

While Fibromyalgia is not covered in this book, the Fibromyalgia patient is advised to have immediate blood tests and a hair analysis done to determine if "sodium fluoride" poisoning is the cause. If fluoride is found then all toothpastes, mouth washes, fluoride treatments by the dentist and the use of fluoridated water must be stopped at once. ***Fluoridated water is used in soft drinks and many other commercially produced liquids. This must be taken in consideration if fluoride poisoning is making the patient ill and the patient has no energy. All sources of "sodium fluoride" must be eliminated. ***Ascorbic acid in high dosages will help chelate sodium fluoride (remove from the blood and other tissues). Extra calcium and CoenzymeQ10 also help to detoxify the patient's body. ***The pain relieving combination of magnesium and malic acid has been mentioned in many studies. This nutrient combination is usually used in daily divided dosages, which total 1,200 mg of malic acid and 400 mg of magnesium; 2 tablets at breakfast, lunch and dinner. Some patients have to double this dosage for a while before they see results. ***Holistic therapy options for inflammation can be found throughout this book. Cod liver oil, Bromelain (a digestive enzyme) and Quercetin may further help the Fibromyalgia patient.

# Chapter III Discussion of Holistic Therapy Options

## Why nutrition instead of medicine?

The known side effects of drugs commonly used for the treatment of connective tissue disease should encourage the reader to investigate natural therapy as an alternative to orthodox medicine and certainly in non-crisis situations. The following list provides information about such drugs:

### Steroids (Corticosteroids)—known side effects

- Osteoporosis
- Cataracts
- Glaucoma
- Ulcers
- Infections
- Fragile skin

### Prednisone

- Depresses the auto-immune system and leaves the patient vulnerable to infections

- Can cause a feeling of "spaciness" or "lightheadedness"
- Can cause problems with patient's memory
- Can cause large weight gain, adding stress to the cardiovascular system

NSAD—no steroidal anti-inflammatory drugs

- Can cause intestinal permeability; changes similar to inflammatory bowel disease
- Can cause NSAD enteropathy; similar to Crohn's disease

# Holistic therapy options

A discussion of essential connective tissue nutrients and how they can be of help

## To strengthen and normalize connective tissue

### MSM—Methylsulfonylmethane

- How taken: granules or tablets
- Daily dosage: 1-2 mg per kg body weight for prevention
- Specific for crisis care: 10-50 mg per kg body weight for acute and chronic cases (kg = about 2 lbs.)

### Tissue Salt #12 Silicea

- This essential nutrient is needed for bone cells, ligament cells, tendon and muscle cells
- Must be supplemented to prevent or treat disease
- Silicea (or Silica) strengthens bone tissue
- Available as sub-lingual tablets. Follow instructions on container; Horsetail tea, a natural source of silica, can also be purchased in all health food stores.

## Tissue Salt #5 Kali. Muriaticum

- Kal. Mur is an essential connective tissue nutrient. In the body it has an attraction for fibrin, a nitrogenous protein. Living tissue cells form a thin covering, called membranes, which normally secrete sufficient fluid to keep nearby tissues moist and supplied with nutrients. If these membranes become inflamed as in connective tissue disease, the cells will benefit from Kal. Mur. Supplementation. Follow directions on container

## Manganese—a trace mineral

- Manganese is essential for the prevention of tendon problems. Example: Hock's disease, a problem often experienced by teenage athletes who go through growth spurts which deplete their manganese levels. Excessive sweating also contributes to such a deficiency. Manganese supplements will help to normalize tendon tissues

## Unsaturated essential fatty acids prevent arthritis-type problems in C.T.D. patients. Natural sources:

- Flax seed oils and other seed oils
- Evening Primrose oil
- Borage oil
- Fish liver oils

## Ascorbic acid (vitamin C)

- Ascorbic acid is an essential nutrient to prevent scurvy and sub-scurvy symptoms and is needed for all rheumatic disease categories, including the connective tissue diseases (collagen diseases). Ascorbic acid is needed to produce collagen, the cellular glue which holds connective tissue together
- Dr Linus Pauling, famous vitamin C researcher and many other scientists have reported that the human body does not store vitamin C. Therefore it must be supplied from the

food we eat. They also stated that the human body requires at least 10,000 mg of vitamin C daily to maintain healthy cells. The modern diet however is so very low in vitamin C that very few people ever get enough. The direct result of vitamin C deficiency can be seen in connective tissue disease; many of the symptoms of this disease indicate a severe and chronic deficiency which must be corrected to make any kind of progress. Ascorbic acid (vitamin C) is best taken in divided dosages throughout the day and best tolerated in the esterified form, labeled as "Ester C". This type of vitamin has a neutral ph and is easily assimilated and well tolerated.

## Kelp—sea vegetation

- Kelp contains important trace minerals which help to overcome sudden numbness, tingling and especially the extreme inner coldness many C.T.D. patients experience when vasospasms occur. Iodine found in Kelp helps to normalize thyroid function

# Holistic therapy options

## Natural antibiotic substances

Natural substances which have anti-viral, anti-bacterial and anti-fungal action:

- Colloidal silver in liquid form, taken internally
- Colloidal silver crème—applied to skin
- Ascorbic acid (vitamin C)
- Ascorbic acid crème—applied to skin
- Acidophilus and other bacilli strains
- Alfalfa (all parts of the plant)
- Aloe Vera gel and liquid
- Apply cider vinegar (unfiltered)
- Bioflavonoid family and other flavones
- Cayenne—can be used instead of penicillin and works well with ascorbic acid
- DMG (Dimethylglycine) formerly known as B15 or Pangamic acid—tablet or capsule
- Echinacea—leaves and root
- Garlic—best raw
- Goldenseal—short term use only

- Honey—raw, unheated
- Honey comb—one tablespoon chewed for ten minutes; then dispose of wax
- Pau d'arco bark—especially for Candida
- Propolis (bee product)
- Red Clover tea
- Reishi mushroom
- Rhubarb root
- Royal jelly (bee product)
- Shitake mushroom
- Combination formulas with anti-fungal and anti-viral action are available in all health food stores.
- An Amish remedy consists of cayenne, ginger, Echinacea, vitamin A and vitamin C.

# Holistic therapy options

## Natural substances to fight infections and inflammations

### How to fight back with natural substances

- Colloidal silver, liquid and crème
- Ascorbic acid and Rose hips
- Aloe Vera, gel and liquid
- Bromelain enzyme—anti-inflammatory
- Chlorophyll
- DMG (Dimethylglycine)
- Evening Primrose oil—anti-inflammatory
- Garlic (powerful antibiotic against bacteria, viruses and fungal problems)
- Propolis (bee product)
- Proteolytic enzymes—anti-inflammatory
- Spleen extract (raw)
- Thymus gland extract (raw)
- Zinc tablets or lozenges

# Holistic therapy options

## How to strengthen the immune system

These natural substances are very helpful:

- Ascorbic acid
- Zinc
- Vitamin A and all carotoid nutrients
- Burdock root—stimulates immune system
- Chaparral—radical cell scavenger
- CoenzymeQ10
- Colloidal silver
- DMG (Dimethylglycine)—strengthens both branches of the immune system)
- Echinacea—freeze dried is most effective
- Vitamin E mixed tocopherol
- Garlic—best raw
- Ginseng
- Goldenseal (short-term use only. Long time uses disturbs intestinal flora)
- Red Clover and Chaparral combined

- Reishi mushroom
- Rose hips
- Shitake mushroom

# Holistic therapy options

## Natural anti-inflammatory and pain-reducing substances

These natural substances are of importance:

- Ascorbic acid—very important anti-inflammatory and natural anti-histamine action; helps to reduce pain
- Evening Primrose oil—contains GLA (Gamma Linoleic Acid). Reduces the production of "interleukin1" a substance produced by the white blood cells. GLA converts to two substances, which in turn reduce interleukin1 production by as much as 30%.
- Garlic—high in sulfur and magnesium; ideal anti-inflammatory
- Ginkgo Biloba—100% effective in a study on "Arteritis", the inflammation of the arteries of lower limbs
- Tissue salt #8 Mag. Phos.—anti-spasmodic; indicated in cramping, darting, shooting and spasmodic pain
- Tissue salt #4 Ferr. Phos.—for pain caused by inflammation and throbbing pain

- MSM (Methylsulfonylmethane)—macro-nutrient for the repair of muscles, tendons, ligaments, cartilage, connective tissue, hormones, enzymes and immunoglobulin. Used with tremendous success by veterinarians and—unofficially—by many other physicians as a natural anti-inflammatory substance for bursitis, connective tissue disease and for the prevention and treatment of "Myositis". By reducing inflammation, pain is lessened. For C.T.D. patients with "Synovitis" the combination of Glucosamine Sulphate and MSM can result in dramatic pain relief and reduction of other symptoms. MSM is also beneficial for the central nervous system
- Proteolytic enzymes—provide powerful anti-inflammatory and anti-viral benefits
- Boswelia—a natural anti-inflammatory substance which reduces swelling, redness, pain in joints and counteracts loss of function
- Bromelain—anti-inflammatory substance; reduces pain
- Comfrey poultice (only used externally). This is how: mash in blender a handful of Comfrey leaves with a bit of water. Apply thick pulp to inflamed area. Cover with several thicknesses of flannel. Then wrap Saran wrap around to warm poultice and to prevent seepage. Leave on for two hours. Remove, wash area with water, air dry and let area rest for two hours. Then repeat process, until swelling, redness and pain are reduced.
- Corn silk tea—corn silk contains Malic acid which is used for pain
- Tissue salt #12 Silicea—stomach pain
- Arnica Montana—a homeopathic medicine
- Catnip tea enemas—to reduce high fever and pain caused by inflammation
- Nettle—well-known natural anti-inflammatory remedy
- Huckleberries—best for external application (poultice) to ease inflammation and pain
- Echinacea—for acute inflammation of Scleroderma with

swelling of glands and lymph. Freeze dried powder is most effective taken every two hours; then decrease according to need

- Yerbamate—stimulates natural Cortisone production and has anti-inflammatory action
- Yucca—great natural anti-inflammatory action to reduce pain in C.D.T. patients

# Holistic Therapy Options

## Natural pain fighters for bones, muscles, ligaments, tendons, lymph system and glands

### Bones

- Silicea Tissue salt #12—needed for normal bone cell formation. Sublingual tablets
- Tissue salt #8 Mag. Phos.—needed for pain and cramps
- Tissue salt #4 Ferr. Phos.—needed for all emergencies
- Mezotrace, a complete mineral supplement which contains all gross and trace minerals including silver, gold, germanium, copper and boron. This supplement also provides balanced amounts of magnesium and calcium
- Glucosamine Sulphate—very important nutrient for the restoration of bone density. This form of Glucosamine is much more easily assimilated and has shown to be effective in reducing pain in the C.T.D. patient

Muscles—Nutrients needed to prevent or treat cramping

- Calcium—for normal contraction and relaxation of

muscles

- Magnesium—same
- Vitamin E d-alpha—increases oxygen uptake and improves circulation
- Ginkgo Biloba—essential for peripheral circulation
- CoenzymeQ10—increases oxygen and circulation
- Niacin—helps to relax and open arteries and prevent cramping
- Chamomile tea—relaxes muscles. Long term use is not advisable
- Chaparral leaves—tea used for leg cramps
- Ginger roots and rhizomes—prevents leg cramps
- Scullcap—prevents leg cramps
- Tissue salt #8 Mag. Phos.—prevents cramping
- Valerian root—very relaxing; promotes sleep and muscle relaxation

### Muscles—to prevent or treat muscle spasms

- Celery seeds
- Ginger roots and rhizomes
- Licorice roots (contraindicated in high blood pressure)
- Scullcap
- Valerian root
- Vitamin E d-alpha
- Calcium lactate
- Tissue salt #8 Mag. Phos.—relaxes muscles

### Muscles—to prevent or treat muscle inflammation

- Ginkgo Biloba
- Evening Primrose oil (GLA)
- MSM (see natural anti-inflammatory remedies)
- Proteolytic enzymes
- Boswelia
- Chickweed
- Comfrey (external use only)
- Corn silk

- Catnip
- Nettle
- Echinacea
- Yucca
- Yerbamate—stimulates natural Cortisone production
- White Oak—contains sulfur; also found in MSM and Echinacea
- Tissue salt #4 Ferr. Phos.—indicated in all inflammations

### Ligaments and tendons—to strengthen and repair

- B6 (Pyridoxine)
- Ascorbic acid
- Manganese—a trace mineral
- Tissue salt #4 Ferr. Phos.—sprains and strains

### For all pain in bones, muscles, tendons and ligaments

- Germanium—a trace mineral
- MSM—use instead of Aspirin
- Capsaicin in pepper—works like aspirin. First patient feels worse, then better
- Malic acid and magnesium combination supplement
- Glucosamine sulphate
- Corn silk—contains malic acid which reduces pain
- Arnica Montana (homeopathic remedy)

### To prevent hardening of tissue in Scleroderma

- Vitamin E d-alpha tocopherol
- Ascorbic acid (vitamin C)—needed in high amounts; 10-15 grams daily in divided dosages to chelate out toxic metals and other harmful substances and to aggressively stimulate the lymph system into better function

### Glandular and lymph swelling and inflammation

- Echinacea, freeze-dried powder every two hours. Decrease when improved. Tincture does not work as well because of

alcohol contents. Echinacea contains sulfur, a natural anti-inflammatory substance which reduces swelling
- Mullein tea—decreases swelling and pain
- Tissue salt #4 Ferr. Phos.—anti-inflammatory
- Tissue salt #5 Kali. Mur.—swollen glands

## Pain relief for Rheumatoid Arthritis, Osteoarthritis and Rheumatism

- Boswelia—natural anti-inflammatory for swelling, redness and joint pain
- MSM—anti-inflammatory, reduces pain
- Glucosamine sulphate—works as well or better than Tylenol. Works well for osteoarthritis
- Celery seeds—for arthritis
- Catnip tea—for arthritis
- Chamomile tea—for rheumatism (no long-term use)
- Chaparral leaves—for leg pain
- Licorice root—best for skeletal muscle spasms (do not take when high blood pressure is a problem)
- Yerbamate tea—for arthritis
- Yucca—for arthritis
- Scullcap—for pain relief
- Chrysanthemum tea—for headaches occurring in arthritis, osteoarthritis or rheumatism
- Tissue salt #4 Ferr. Phos.—pain relief
- Tissue salt #8 Mag. Phos—pain relief

# Discussion of holistic therapy options

## The role of ascorbic acid in

Connective Tissue Diseases (Collagen Diseases), Rheumatoid Arthritis, Osteoarthritis and Rheumatism

Many research statistics identify arthritis, rheumatism and related rheumatic conditions as "collagen diseases" and the involvement of "collagen protein". High ascorbic acid levels are essential in order to synthesize high quality collagen and to continually maintain this quality. When a deficiency develops, either collagen protein synthesis stops altogether, or causes poor quality protein production. This results in weakened and abnormal tissues. The deficiency creates bone and joint effects which fall into the category of "clinical scurvy". Abnormalities in collagen protein are the reason for crippling deformities, associated with rheumatic disease and other congenital connective tissue defects. ***Rinehart and coworkers wrote in 1930-1938 that "deficiencies of ascorbic acid plus an infection are responsible for the rheumatoid process". It was stated further that "rheumatic fever is caused by a major ascorbic acid deficiency". ***Other contributing factors to consider are malnutrition, the effect of weather-climate changes, geographical distribution, age at time of illness and stress. This research further showed that there are symptomatic similarities between rheumatic fever and latent scurvy. The researchers conclude "that infection alone does not cause connective tissue disease, but the combination of infection and gross ascorbic acid deficiency does". ***In later years a vast number of experiments were done with ascorbic acid, only to be discontinued because researchers could not duplicate the wonderful results of earlier colleagues. They were trying to simply correct a nutritional deficiency using fairly small amounts of ascorbic acid (something which is still done today by many physicians), when they should have been treating a serious disease with very large amounts of this essential nutrient. To just raise the blood level to normal is simply not enough. The blood level must reach mega-scorbic levels (saturation levels) in the very ill person to achieve an improvement or cure.

Summary: Ascorbic acid must be provided at megascorbic levels to have a definite therapeutic effect on collagen diseases. It has been suggested that in acute or chronic cases six to ten grams administered through an I.V. are successful in providing anti-rheumatic activity; but it is better to provide even higher amounts if tolerated well. In one case listed by researchers a patient suffering from rheumatic fever was given from one to ten grams ascorbic acid daily. Rapid improvement followed with complete recovery in three to four weeks. *** Dr. W. Shute's vitamin E research is equally important to all patients with rheumatic fever.

# Holistic Therapy Options

## Natural vasodilators

Especially important for patients with Raynaud's phenomenon or Raynaud's disease who are at risk for gangrene, stroke or suffering from high blood pressure

Specific therapeutic nutrients which help to protect heart and blood vessels

D.M.G. (Dimethylglycine), also known as B15, Pangamic acid

- Prevents major strokes if taken regularly and especially after a T.I.A. episode, which is usually a warning sign of a more serious stroke to come.
- Prevents T.I.A.'s (minor strokes)
- Carries oxygen, therefore improves tissue oxygenation
- Prevents leg ulceration
- Prevents gangrene
- Combined with vitamin E d-alpha, restores normal blood flow to the brain

## Germanium

- Improves tissue oxygenation. Suggested daily dose 200 mg

## Choline and Inositol combination

- Helps to improve circulation
  CoenzymeQ10
- In dosages above 120 mg daily improves tissue oxygenation. This nutrient has proven to be of tremendous help to congestive heart failure patients; in doses of 380 mg daily or more it helps to normalize the body in all chronic diseases

## M.S.M. (Methylsulfonylmethane)

- Enhances circulation

## Niacin and Niacinamide

- Dilate arteries. Niacin in single very large doses is harmful to the liver. Some medical physicians have prescribed doses as high as 5,000 mg daily to lower cholesterol. However, this creates a huge imbalance with other B-vitamins and can cause hepatitis-type symptoms. Please, consult health food store counselor about correct dosage

## Ascorbic acid

- Improves tissue oxygenation and blood flow
  Bioflavonoids (belong to the ascorbic acid complex)
- Strengthen capillary and vein walls (e.g. in varicose veins)
- Help to prevent bleeding episodes (e.g. nose bleed)
- A highly effective form of bioflavonoid is "Pycnogenol"

## Vitamin E d-alpha tocopherol

- Carries oxygen
- Prevents clotting, and especially in the emulsified form dissolves fresh blood clots in the lungs, legs and heart

- Improves circulation through oxygenation
- Acts as a natural anti-coagulant (blood thinner)
- Helps overcome angina pain
- Repairs blood vessel damage
- Builds natural by-passes in the heart after an infarct
- Treats intermittent claudication
- Very important for Raynaud's patients, since it helps to prevent gangrene and treats existing gangrene (see Dr. W. Shute's research)

### GLA found in salmon, cod, and mackerels but also in Canola and Flaxseed oils

- Lowers triglycerides
- Prevents blood platelets from sticking together

### Chromium—a trace mineral

- Lowers triglycerides

### Superoxide Dismutase (S.O.D.)

- Prevents gangrene
- Greatly improves circulation
- Greatly improves oxygenation and blood flow

### Lecithin

- Lowers blood fats
- Lowers blood cholesterol

### Bromelain

- Lowers cholesterol
- Treats fibrin clots in varicose veins
- Treats intermittent claudication
- Improves warmth of legs by more than 50%
- Is helpful in treating ulcerous lesions (100%)

### Tissue salt #4 Ferr. Phos

- Acts as an oxygen carrier

### All B-vitamins

- Needed in high dosages to protect the nervous system, nerve sheaths, and brain function and to protect against tendon and ligament problems. B6, B3 and Folate also help lower cholesterol

## Natural Vasodilators—Herbal Helpers

### Ginkgo Biloba –one capsule three times daily

- Increases peripheral circulation
- Dilates arteries, veins and capillaries
- Helpful in cerebral insufficiency
- Counteracts arterial leg disease
- Greatly improves lower limb circulation
- Treats other vascular disorders
- Very effectively treats blood vessel spasms
- Can improve peripheral pain by over 50%
- Studies show it improves blood flow in Scleroderma
- Helpful in "diabetic micro-angiopathy"
- Helpful in "acrocyanosis" a circulatory condition which leaves hands and feet cold, blue and sweaty
- Ginkgo Biloba in phytosome form is especially helpful to strengthen the immune system
- Ginkgo combined with Choline benefits Raynaud's patients and increases endurance in walking, enhances memory, improves memory loss problems and improves brain function through better circulation, oxygenation and blood flow
- Normalizes blood pressure

### Hawthorn berry extract –berries and tincture are used

- Carries oxygen, dilates blood vessels of the heart

- Restores blood vessel interior walls
- Lowers cholesterol
- Relieves and helps manage angina pain
- Prevents angina pain
- Prevents heart vessel spasms
- Benefits heart disease patients

## Butcher's broom

- Carries oxygen and enhances circulation
- Prevents leg cramps

Other herbal vasodilators

- Cayenne—oxygen carrier; improves circulation
- Pau d'Arco—oxygen carrier
- Ginseng—helps to normalize blood pressure
- Black Cohosh—reduces blood pressure and cholesterol
- Blessed Thistle—improves circulation and heart function
- Blue Cohosh—helps with low blood pressure problems
- Corn silk—lowers blood pressure; natural diuretic
- Gotu Kola –helps blood pressure and congestive heart failure
- Fenugreek seeds—lower cholesterol
- Scullcap—improves circulation; strengthens heart
- Thyme—lowers cholesterol
- Uva Ursi—strengthens heart muscle
- Valerian Root—improves circulation; natural sedative
- Wood Betony—strengthens heart

Cautions: always purchase herbs from a legitimate source. Always discuss plans to include herbs with your N.D., M.D. or pharmacist. Herbs are a natural source of important medicines and must be used according to established guidelines.

## Natural vasodilators—plant helpers

Garlic is most effective when used raw

- Prevents clotting and platelets from sticking together
- Natural anti-coagulant/blood thinner
- Lowers high blood pressure, cholesterol and triglycerides

- Strengthens blood vessels
- Helps with arteriosclerosis

Green juices from leafy vegetables—enhance blood flow
Celery—lowers blood pressure
Dandelion leaves and roots—natural diuretic
Watercress—natural diuretic; relieves edema

Miscellaneous vasodilator therapy

hot foot bath for 5 minutes, alternate with 2 minutes of cold foot bath. Repeat three to four times daily until improved; then once daily

# Holistic Therapy Options

Natural antioxidants

- Ginkgo Biloba
- Ascorbic acid (vitamin C)
- CoenzymeQ10
- Zinc
- Selenium
- Vitamin E, in the d-alpha and mixed tocopherol form
- Beta Carotene and all other carotoids which are found in red, yellow and green vegetables and fruit
- B6 (Pyridoxine)
- Cysteine and Methionine (amino acids)
- S.O.D. (Superoxide Dismutase)
- Tissue salt #4 Ferr. Phos.

# Holistic Therapy Options

---

## Natural therapy for skin conditions

Horsetail stems contain silica for skin, nails and hair

- Please, use in the form of Silica tissue salt #12 or Horsetail tea purchased from a health food store or herbalist. Do not self-treat with self-collected plant
- Heals connective tissue
- Increases calcium assimilation

Evening Primrose oil—contains GLA; heals skin
Flaxseed oil—contains essential fatty acids for skin
Vitamin E oil—improves skin circulation, elasticity
Aloe Vera—wonderful skin nutrient and antiseptic
Ginkgo Biloba—helps Scleroderma patients
Emu oil—heals skin

## For chronic viral or bacterial skin eruptions Natural antiseptic therapy options

- Ascorbic acid—mix with water; apply several times daily
- Silver crème—apply as needed
- Aloe Vera—apply several times daily

- Apple cider vinegar—2 tbsp. in ¼ c. water—apply often
- Lemon juice—apply often; a natural antiseptic

## Natural anti-microbial therapy

- Raw honey—apply externally to affected areas; also one teaspoon of honey taken internally several times daily

Poultices for skin inflammations and sores using a strong tea prepared from one of the following choices. (External only)

- Chrysanthemum tea poultice
- Burdock root tea poultice
- Coltsfoot tea poultice
- Comfrey—mix leaves and a little water to make thick mash; apply to inflammation; cover with old towel; wrap saran wrap around towel; leave on for two hours, remove and wash with clear water; let area rest for two hours, then repeat process, until inflammation has subsides. Use Comfrey for external application only. Do not drink Comfrey tea. It contains a harmful alkaloid.
- Hawthorn berries tea poultice
- Red Clover tea poultice
- Red Raspberry tea poultice
- Chamomile tea poultice

## Vitiligo in the connective tissue disease patient

Connective tissue diseases produce loss of pigment in many patients. In some, the pigmentation is lost in large skin areas, while others have only very minor changes. The following nutrients have shown to be effective in the treatment of Vitiligo, but do not offer any guarantee that full pigmentation will occur. But, it is worth a try....

- Tyrosine (amino acid)
- B6 (Pyridoxine)
- PABA (Para-aminobenzoic acid, a B vitamin)
- B5 (Pantothenic acid, a B vitamin)

## Skin discolorations

- Dandelion—use milky extract from stem
- Ascorbic acid—counteracts premature aging of skin
- "Reviva"—a natural skin lightener product

## Itching

Itching is experienced by many C.T.D. patients and is usually caused by nutritional deficiencies which cause irritation and possible scarring of nerve endings (such as in shingles)

- Apply vitamin E oil over pain area; also take vitamin E supplements
- If itching is due to kidney malfunction: increase water intake; try potassium supplement
- Indicates a vitamin A and/or potassium deficiency

## Allergenic itching

- ascorbic acid to help the adrenal glands which are the anti-itch glands

Itchy eyes—indicates a vitamin A deficiency

## Vaginal itching

- Common in C.T.D. patients with Candida. Such infections can be treated topically with colloidal silver or Aloe Vera.
- Some itching may be due to ph imbalances. If the body is too acid, vaginal and rectal itching can occur. Coffee, smoking and alcohol must be avoided.
- Carrot juice is very effective in balancing ph acidity or alkalinity and reduces or eliminates itching

## Burning sensations

- Burning sensations in the feet and hands are often experienced by C.T.D. patients. Usually this can be explained with "overactive nerve endings".

- Tissue salt #6 Kali. Phos. May be helpful
- Usually a B1 deficiency which responds to supplementation
- If hands and feet experience burning sensations vitamin B1 and Pantothenic acid can be supplemented to correct the situation.

# Holistic Therapy Options

## Natural insomnia fighters

### Natural tranquilizers and sedatives

Natural nutrients and various herbs for insomnia which also have a calming and tranquilizing effect can provide much desired and safe relief to patients, who have trouble going to sleep, remaining asleep and those who have trouble relaxing

- Ginger—has tranquilizing effect
- St. John's Wort—natural tranquilizer
- Thyme—mildly tranquilizing
- Valerian root—used for relaxation, insomnia and sedation
- Celery seed—has a sedative effect
- Chamomile—acts as a nerve tonic; calming effect
- Garlic—induces sleep
- Hops flowers and stems—combat nervousness and insomnia
- Scullcap—induces and aids sleep
- L-Tryptophan—acts as sedative

- Calcium lactate—acts as a sedative
- Warm milk plus 1 tbsp. raw honey—sedative effect

# Holistic Therapy Options

## Glandular nutrients

- Ginkgo Biloba improves function of reproductive organs, especially when male patients are on high blood pressure medication and become impotent as a side effect of the medication
- Zinc combined with Damiane and Saw Palmetto may help erratic impotence
- Yerbamate tea stimulates natural Cortisone production in the adrenal glands
- Alfalfa tea improves function of the pituitary gland
- Bladder wrack improves function of the thyroid gland
- Kelp, which contains iodine, improves thyroid function
- Chaparral leaves improve absorption of ascorbic acid by the adrenal glands
- Dong Quai roots improve vaginal dryness and help the ovaries and testes through hormone-like action
- Ginseng strengthens the adrenal glands; it also stimulates male sex glands to overcome impotence
- Kotu Kola seeds, nuts and roots stimulate reproductive glands

- Irish moss contains iodine and helps to corrects thyroid problems, including the development of goiter
- Licorice root stimulates the adrenal glands and has an estrogen-like hormonal effect. However, this substance must not be used by patients with high blood pressure
- Lobelia aids in hormone production
- Parsley is beneficial for the thyroid
- Red Raspberry bark, leaves and roots strengthen the uterus and other female organs; also known to alleviate childbirth pain
- Rose hips—fruit nourishes the adrenal glands because of its high vitamin C content
- Sarsaparilla helps to overcome impotence
- Uva Ursi is beneficial for the female patient for correction of female disorders

# Holistic Therapy Options

## To counteract stress and calm the body

### Helpful nutrients and herbs:

- Chamomile tea calms and relaxes
- Hops flowers tea calm and relax
- Valerian root tea or capsules calm, relax and help the patient to sleep
- St. John's Wort tea or capsules relax, help depression and help patients to sleep better
- Entire B vitamin complex is important for the nervous system. These nutrients nourish nerve tissue and help patients to better deal with stress. Individual B vitamins play an important role in various neuroses, phobias and panic disorders
- Calcium, magnesium and potassium help to stabilize the nervous system, relax muscles and help the patient to build up resistance to stress. All dried legumes, such as beans, lentils and peas provide high amounts of these nerve minerals

- A diet high in ascorbic acid plus supplementation is equally important for C.T.D. patients. This essential nutrient is needed for all body cells, but especially important for normal adrenal gland function and to prevent depletion
- L-Tryptophan is a natural sedative. Both milk and honey contain L-Trytophan. That is why warm milk mixed with honey makes a great bedtime drink to relax the nerves and muscles

# Holistic Therapy Options

Nutrients and herbs for the mind and brain tissues

- Choline (B vitamin) helps to restore memory
- CoenzymeQ10 increases oxygen supply to the brain, improves circulation and aids the memory
- Lecithin improves memory
- Ginkgo Biloba increases blood and oxygen flow to the brain; prevents and treats any dementia; has the potential to treat and/or prevent Alzheimer's; helps to overcome short-term memory loss
- To prevent suicidal tendency—magnesium is a potent anti-stress nutrient and protects against suicidal thoughts and depression. Magnesium is a very important nutrient for all chronically ill people
- B1 (Thiamine) aids in preventing memory loss and trouble concentrating
- D.M.G. (Dimethylglycine) combined with vitamin E increases blood flow, protects against strokes and resulting brain damage and mental deterioration
- Schizophrenia-type symptoms are helped with ascorbic

acid and B6

- Entire B vitamin complex nourishes the nervous system and helps patient to maintain a positive outlook
- Zinc is usually deficient in patients who exhibit aggression and rage. Such patients may have very high copper levels and benefit from zinc to offset the effect
- Vitamin E d-alpha tocopherol—oxygenates brain

# Holistic Therapy Options for spinal nerves, bones, ligaments, tendons, muscles and synovial membranes

---

### Herbs and specific nutrients for repair and healing of damaged tissues

- M.S.M. (Methylsulfonylmethane)
- Glucosamine Sulphate which is more easily assimilated than Glucosamine Chondroitin
- B6 provides an important enzyme for forming gamma-aminotutyric acid
- Tissue salt #12 Silica—important for surface of bones

### To stimulate the central nervous system

- Goldenseal
- Gotu Kola

### To provide energy for the muscles

- Iron supplements and food high in iron
- Tissue salt #1 Calc. Fluor.—aids muscles

### To restore bone density

- Calcium
- Glucosamine sulphate
- M.S.M.
- Boron (trace element)
- Tissue salt #12 Silica

### To prevent muscle cramping and to help prevent unwanted calcium deposits in muscle and other tissues

- Magnesium
- Tissue salt #8 Mag. Phos.

### To keep tendons and ligaments flexible and strong and to help repair damaged tissue

- Manganese
- Glucosamine sulphate
- M.S.M.
- Zinc

### To facilitate healing of injured tissue and to strengthen the immune system

- Zinc which is especially needed for bone strength, formation of dense cell structures; to overcome weak tissues; very important for cartilage and ligaments
- Ascorbic acid
- Tissue salt #4 Ferr. Phos.
- M.S.M.
- Glucosamine sulphate

### For normal development of bone cells and cartilage cells

- Perma canaliculus, which contains Chondroitin Sulphate

### For healing and to protect the immune system

- Shark cartilage is used by Chinese healers. However, for the healing of injured vertebrae and resulting nerve damage Glucosamine sulphate and M.S.M. are more readily assimilated and accelerate the healing process

### For brain and spinal cord health

- Kelp tablets and all sea vegetation rich in trace minerals
- Alfalfa roots reach deep into the soil to extract needed and provide important trace minerals
- Colloidal mineral supplement (liquid)

# Holistic Therapy Options

## Neurology

### Nerve nutrients for numbness, tingling and other unusual sensations

- Numbness in arms and legs—B1 and B12
- Numbness in the fingers—B1, B6, B12 and Kelp
- Intermittent numbness—B12 (injection in liquid form or as a spray)
- Tingling feeling in extremities or body—Kelp; calcium
- Local numbness—Biotin; magnesium
- Feelings of bugs crawling on skin or through hair—the entire vitamin B complex is needed in potent dosages
- Phantom pains, which are shooting pains in various body areas—entire vitamin B complex and potassium
- Entire B vitamin complex is very important for all physical and mental stress situations. The sicker a person is, the more ascorbic acid, magnesium, B vitamins and other minerals are needed.
- Creeping sensations on the skin combined with numbness and coldness of extremities—Tissue salt #2 Calc. Phos.

# Holistic Therapy Options
## Urinary system problems

Many things can and often do go wrong with the kidneys and other parts of the urinary system. The reader is advised to look up the "Lupus" section, where extremely detailed entries for various conditions have been listed in the "special help section for the kidneys". ***Patients must seek immediate professional help if sudden or severe pain develops, the urine is very cloudy, or urine production slows down suddenly or stops altogether. These are crisis situations which demand immediate medical care. Once the crisis is past, herbs and supportive nutrients can and should be used to prevent further problems. ***In mild to moderate cases herbal teas can be used to relieve the condition. But it cannot be emphasized enough that kidney problems experienced by a C.T.D. patient must be evaluated and monitored by a medical or a naturopathic physician. ***It is also of the utmost importance, that self-treatment with herbs should not be undertaken without professional advice. Only experienced herbalists, naturopathic physicians or homeopaths are qualified to prescribe specific dosages. Some herbal teas cannot be taken for long periods of time or might conflict with current prescriptions. When planning to combine herbs with present medications the attending physician or pharmacist should be informed of such plans.

# Holistic Therapy Options Preventive nutrients for cancer and radiation damage

## Breast cancer

- High fiber diet
- High dosages of ascorbic acid supplements
- Flaxseed oil
- Soybean oil
- Virgin Olive oil
- Vitamin A, C and E supplements and daily food intake high in these nutrients
- Diet must be high in Beta Carotene and all other carotids (all green, yellow and red vegetables and fruit)

## Stomach cancer

- Eliminate all products containing sodium chloride (commercial salt)
- Use sea salt or vegetable salt instead

## Skin Cancer

- Diet must be high in fresh fruit and vegetables

- Supplementation with high dosage ascorbic acid
- Use of an ascorbic acid solution (water and vitamin C) as a protective sun screen. Vitamin C crème is also of value

## Radiation and chemotherapy effect—how to protect against and to treat naturally

- Bee pollen
- Fennel tea
- Ginseng root
- Kelp leaves

## Radiation burns

- Aloe Vera gel application around the clock. Aloe Vera appears to be extremely successful in treating radiation burns. It has been said that Aloe Vera is the only substance effective for radiation burns

## To inhibit cancer cells

- Suma
- Diet high in fruit and vegetables
- D.M.G.
- Daily intake of supplements and food totaling at least 10,000 mg ascorbic acid
- Combination of vitamin E mixed tocopherol and Selenium daily for anti-oxidant protection
- Daily zinc supplement for anti-oxidant protection
- Daily CoenzymeQ10 supplement for anti-oxidant protection. Use 400 mg daily for active cancer
- Daily Ginkgo-Biloba supplement for anti-oxidant protection
- Daily use of Flaxseed oil in salads, soups and other dishes. Do not heat oil. Add after cooking is complete

## Anti-tumor protection

- Parsley has been effective and can be used daily fresh or

dried in salads, soups and other food
- High ascorbic acid supplement and diet
- D.M.G.
- Ginkgo Biloba

## To fight active cancer

- Red Clover and Chaparral combination tea
- Jonathan Winter herbal tea
- Essiac tea
- Very high ascorbic acid supplementation
- Daily fresh pressed juices from organic vegetables and fruit
- Whole fruit and whole vegetable supplements
- Daily water intake must be 2 quarts
- Daily 1 tbsp. Flaxseed oil plus liberal use of other seed oils such as sunflower and sesame seed oil
- CoEnzymeQ10—400 mg daily in divided dosages

# Holistic Therapy Options
# Eye and vision problems

---

## The role of ascorbic acid and other key nutrients and herbs

### For all eye conditions

- Eyebright; tea or tincture. Use for daily eye wash. Clears eyes of cellular debris; relieves eye strain
- Fennel berries, roots, stems and fruit—use for eye wash
- Fenugreek seeds—strengthens eye

### Dry eye—a symptom of Sjoegren's syndrome

- B6 is essential for normal tear production
- Ascorbic acid is involved in tear-fluid production. Dry eye can be corrected with sufficient ascorbic acid

### Sight problems—Night blindness

- Vitamin A supplement
- Diet high in vitamin A food, such as carrots, yellow fruit, yellow vegetables, fish oil and fish high in vitamins A and D (e.g. Sardines, Mackerel)

Retina—to prevent premature aging and maintain good sight into old age. A chronic ascorbic acid and zinc deficiency contribute to early sight loss or premature aging

- Zinc supplement and food high in zinc
- Bilberry products
- Food high in Lutein
- Optimum ascorbic acid food intake

### Floaters; dark spots before the eye; fluttering sight

- Floaters or sight problems often occur after heavy sugar use and Candida flare-up and improve, when the body has rid itself of the excess sugar. Please, have blood sugar level tested
- Tissue salt #8 Mag. Phos.

### Drooping of eye lids

- Tissue salt #6 Kali. Phos.
- Tissue salt #8 Mag. Phos.
- B6 and potassium, if edema is the cause

### Glaucoma

- To prevent Glaucoma the intraocular pressure must be kept low. Suggested is this: Absolute minimum of 500 mg ascorbic acid daily to prevent blindness. Irvin Stone in his book "Vitamin C and you" states, that 2000 mg daily result in a drop of pressure in Glaucoma

### Deep corneal ulcers

- 1,500 mg ascorbic acid daily (minimum)

### To recover from burns to the eyes

- 1500 mg ascorbic acid daily (minimum)

## Twitching of eye lids

- Tissue salt #6 Kali. Phos.
- Tissue salt #8 Mag. Phos.
- Magnesium 500 mg twice daily

## Diabetic retinopathy

- Vitamin E d-alpha tocopherol 400 IU minimum
- Ascorbic acid 1,500—2,000 mg daily minimum

## Detachment of retina

- High ascorbic acid supplementation

## Cataracts

- High ascorbic acid supplementation to build up cells
- B2 (Riboflavin) deficiency has been identified as a contributing cause
- Older models Microwave ovens caused a dramatic increase in cataracts
- Uveitis can cause cataracts
- Physical and chemical injuries can cause cataracts

## Neuralgia pain in eyes

- Tissue salt #9 Nat. Mur.
- Tissue salt #8 Mag. Phos.
- B12 injections or B12 sublingual drops (very important for patients suffering from Trigeminal Neuralgia)

## Additional information

The role of ascorbic acid in eye health

Ascorbic acid is involved in twelve different biochemical processes and appears to play a role in the following conditions:

- Diabetic retinopathy
- Detachment of the retina
- Maintenance of proper fluid consistency (see Sjoegren's section)

Dryness, a gritty feeling and an irritation of the eye as well as an irritation at the entrance to the esophagus can be improved with increased ascorbic acid levels. Both symptoms are common complaints with C.T.D. patients. And, as stated before, a person diagnosed with Lupus may also experience Sjoegren's syndrome and/or Raynaud's phenomenon symptoms. ***The ascorbic acid content of the eyes is higher in percentage than that of the blood or other tissues. Therefore, sub-marginal levels of ascorbic acid affect the eyes. The following ascorbic acid levels were established in normal test persons:

- 30% was found in the cornea
- 47-94% in the corneal epithelium
- 34% in the lens; 22% in the retina

In comparison the only other body tissues with higher levels than the eyes are the adrenal glands with 97-160% and the pituitary with 126%. This information clearly indicates the need for consistent supplementation with ascorbic acid to avoid damage to the eyes and other organs of the C.T.D. patient.

# Holistic therapy options For patients who have trouble expelling mucus

To expel mucus from throat and chest and to increase fluidity

- Increase water intake to two quarts daily
- Blue Vervain tea
- Chickweed tea; or fresh in salads
- Fresh lemon juice dissolved in water
- Horehound tea or lozenges

To soothe inflamed mucus membranes and help the healing process

- Buchu tea
- Chickweed tea or fresh in salads
- Chamomile tea. Steam is inhaled.
- Slippery Elm lozenges

# Holistic Therapy Options Prevention and treatment of Cardiovascular problems and the important role of ascorbic acid

There is substantial evidence that sub-marginal levels of ascorbic acid cause chronic scurvy. This in turn results in

- Degenerative lesions on the heart valves
- Degenerative lesions on the heart muscle
- Can contribute to myocardial degeneration
- Can contribute to arteriosclerosis of the lungs, liver, spleen and kidneys
- Capillary rupture and hemorrhages in arterial walls
- Inflammation of heart valves
- Occasional Pericarditis
- Is a factor in coronary thrombosis due to impaired collagen production
- Causes the body to make more cholesterol
- Can contribute to high blood pressure
- Increases the risk of hemorrhages or clots

In one study of 455 adult patients, over half of the patients had subnormal ascorbic acid levels, and of these 81% were coronary patients. ***In a second study, almost two thirds of heart patients and coronary thrombotic patients showed very low ascorbic acid levels. ***Further research showed that old age further aggravates already existing deficiencies and that an existing ascorbic acid deficiency is further complicated by and is increased even more by chronic illness and stress. Several research studies showed that some segments of arteries, which are subjected to mechanical stress, are low in ascorbic acid, while other segments are not. ***In a study done with Guinea pigs depriving the animals of ascorbic acid in their food quickly led to scurvy and the rapid onset of atherosclerosis. When a thrombosis (clot) occurs, it must not be considered a problem in itself, but rather seen as a defense response by the body to make time for the repair of damaged blood vessels. The clot blocks the area to allow time for such repair. ***High blood pressure and the excessive stretching of blood vessels result in rupture and bleeding in the patient with subnormal ascorbic acid levels. The body produces the clot in response. Maintaining high ascorbic acid levels should be used as a protective mechanism. Patients are being encouraged to use a combination of high ascorbic acid dosages plus additional vitamin E d-alpha tocopherol supplementation for consistent protection. It should not be suppressed through the use of anticoagulants with dangerous side effects. The hemorrhage would not occur, if the tissues were made up of high quality collagen. Optimum ascorbic acid intake in the form of fresh food and supplements guarantees healthy and durable tissue. ***The aorta can synthesize cholesterol. An ascorbic acid deficiency causes cholesterol synthesis. The greater the deficiency, the more cholesterol accumulates in the body tissues. Ascorbic acid therefore can reduce cholesterol.

# Discussion of Holistic Therapy Options

## Stroke prevention

The protective role of ascorbic acid and other nutrients

Ascorbic acid

Studies in 1981 showed that large numbers of deaths occur annually just from strokes and that even larger numbers of patients are either totally or partially disabled. And, no doubt these numbers are much higher today. ***It was estimated at the time that at least a million people have had one or even several small strokes. These strokes are called "Transient Ischemic Attack" or T.I.A. During a T.I.A. a small clot passes through the brain and causes temporary problems, which usually disappear within 48-62 hours without permanent damage. Sometimes a person experiencing such a stroke may just momentarily feel slightly nauseous, dizzy or experience slowness of speech, garbled speech, difficulty with walking or a slight paralysis on one side for a few days. ***All research with ascorbic acid confirms that this essential nutrient is very important for the vascular system of the brain. Submarginal levels of ascorbic acid cause asymptomatic chronic vascular damage, until some major part suddenly gives way and massive hemorrhages or thrombi occur. Sub-marginal ascorbic acid levels weaken important structures and lead to strokes. Megascorbic levels can prevent these problems.

The importance of vitamin E d-alpha tocopherol and D.M.G. (Dimethylglycine)

The reader is encouraged to thoroughly study Dr. Wilfred Shute's vitamin E research for cardiovascular health. Vitamin E provides very important protective action against blood clots and is capable of creating vascular by-passes by strengthening smaller blood vessels in the vicinity of a large damaged blood vessel. Vitamin E contributes to the development of new blood vessels. These can form a "natural by-pass".

Very extensive Russian research with D.M.G. (Dimethylglycine) has provided hundreds of important study results, which document the value of this special nutrient for the prevention of T.I.A.'s as well as big strokes. ***A series of small strokes indicates that a big stroke may follow soon and that preventive action must be taken at once. D.M.G. was of great help to the author's husband, when he suffered several T.I.A.'s within one year. Utilizing the Russian research, D.M.G. was used consistently and the feared big stroke never occurred.

# Holistic Therapy Options Natural Candida fighters

All participants in a private study conducted by the author suffered from Candida Albicans and other chronic fungal problems. The reader can use the following suggestions to correct and control Candida and other fungal problems:

- Garlic—a natural antibiotic which also counteracts fungal infections in the intestinal tract. A daily clove of raw garlic is best; many companies produce garlic tablets for those who cannot tolerate fresh garlic
- Acidophilus and other strains of beneficial bacilli are equally important for restoring a normal protective flora. These products are available in powder, liquid and tablet form
- Lab tests should be performed to determine what types of fungal infections are present. A strict anti-yeast diet must be followed, until subsequent testing shows an improvement. A maintenance diet follows which continues to exclude all excessive use of sugar, fermented products, yeast products and any products containing fungi (e.g. mushrooms) and mold (e.g. blue cheese). Exposure to mold and mildew in

the home and other environments must also be avoided to prevent further infections.

Many excellent natural and very specific homeopathic herbal combinations products are widely available. These provide natural substances which will help to restore and then maintain normal flora function.

# Chapter IV
# What patients need to know about certain supplements before beginning a holistic program and how and why these supplements work

When high dosages of ascorbic acid are taken (more than 5,000 mg daily), the entire B-complex and complete mineral supplement plus additional B12, Folate (Folic acid) and magnesium must be supplied. Adult dosages under 5,000 mg are fine as long as the entire B-complex and a complete mineral supplement are taken also. Above 5,000 mg daily: five B12 drops under the tongue twice daily, plus two 400 mcg Folate tablets daily and 500 mg magnesium citrate at least once a day. A liquid B12 formula with Folate is available, which can be used sublingually (under the tongue) for quicker absorption. ***"Ester C" can be taken without concern for acidity, while many other forms of ascorbic acid supplements may prove to be too acid for a sensitive stomach. Because esterified ascorbic acid is bound to minerals and the patient might be taking a mineral supplement plus extra magnesium, it is possible that the body becomes too alkaline. This can be avoided by dissolving 1/8 tsp. of regular ascorbic acid powder in a glass of water. This will provide the necessary acidity to offset the alkalinizing effect o minerals. ***Dosages also depend on body weight and age. Children, toddlers and babies obviously require smaller quantities of nutrients than adults. Also considered must be the fact, that the more seriously ill a person is the more ascorbic acid is needed.

## How and why do these supplements work?

Ascorbic acid crystals and Ester C

- Stimulate collagen production
- Normalize connective tissue
- Repair inferior tissues
- Function as a natural anti-histamine
- Have diuretic action
- Detoxify the body of harmful substances
- Ester C, the esterified form of ascorbic acid, almost triples the action of regular vitamin C. So, when taking two 500 mg Ester C tables its action is close to 3,000 mg of ordinary ascorbic acid. Ester C is more easily assimilated and remains in the body tissues much longer. Because Ester C has a neutral ph; it causes no gastric upsets, even in large amounts

## DMG (Dimethylglycine) also known as B15 and Pangamic acid

- Powerful protector for both branches of the immune system
- Essential nutrient for the prevention of strokes
- Essential nutrient for the prevention of ulceration due to impaired circulation
- Essential nutrient for the prevention of gangrene in Raynaud's phenomenon and Raynaud's disease

## Ginkgo Biloba

- Ginkgo Biloba is an "adaptogen' such as Ginseng
- Vitalizes the brain
- Restores memory
- Improves concentration

- Improves peripheral circulation
- Has been clearly identified as an essential substance to prevent senile dementia and Alzheimer's symptoms
- Has a very great balancing effect on circulation
- Protects the immune system

## Chromium picolinate

- Known as the "glucose tolerance factor"
- Identified as the "master balance for a consistent blood sugar level"
- The "picolinate" form of chromium helps the body to turn fat into muscle tissue
- Important for all patients suffering from fluctuating blood sugar levels

## Bromelain

- Bromelain is a digestive enzyme
- Has natural anti-inflammatory properties
- Reduces pain
- Helps the body to utilize fat

## Acidophilus

- Is used to maintain or restore normal intestinal flora
- Essential for patients suffering from Candida Albicans or other fungal/yeast infections

Additional comments: Dr. Helbing-Sheafe stated in a recent lecture that the amount of pain and general discomfort in C.T.D. patients is directly related to the degree of acute or chronic yeast-fungal infections. Very acute yeast infections result in often unbearable allergy reactions, great pain and other body malfunctions and must be treated naturally and consistently to free the body of this awful stress.

## Magnesium

- Maintains normal electrical impulses to the heart

- Reduces pain
- Very important anti-stress nutrient
- Important to all people suffering from irregular heart beat
- A combination of magnesium and malic acid has proven to be more effective than Ibuprofen in reducing pain in the Fibromyalgia patient
- Magnesium citrate appears to be more potent than other forms of this mineral
- A significant magnesium deficiency has been found in fatal heart attacks
- Magnesium deficiency is extremely common in individuals attempting or committing suicide. Its role as an anti-stress nutrient therefore is significant. Some researchers claim that the high rate of suicide among young individuals is directly related to a gross magnesium deficiency which is caused by eating nutrient-poor food.

  Mezotrace
- A wonderful and complete mineral and trace element supplement which is mined from an ancient sea bed and provides all gross and trace minerals.
- Supplies all the mineral nutrients humans need and never get from their diet
- Taken consistently in recommended dosages it has helped many patients to reduce the pain of arthritis-type illnesses and stabilize their illness
- Its high calcium-magnesium-potassium content makes it an ideal heart and connective tissue supplement

Comments by the author: I have absolutely no connection to the company which produces Mezotrace. However, this product has helped me personally a great deal, and I have taken it consistently for many years. I therefore feel qualified to vouch for its effectiveness.

## Evening Primrose oil

- Essential anti-inflammatory substance

- Involved in healing process

## Vitamin B-complex

- Needed for various central nervous system functions
- A deficiency in biotin, B1 or B6 for instance can cause tingling and numbness
- A deficiency in B5 (Pantothenic acid) can impair adrenal gland function. B5 and ascorbic acid are essential for normal adrenal gland function

Additional comments: It is impossible to list the functions of all B-vitamins in this paper; however, it is important to say that connective tissue disease affects the assimilation and absorption of food. C.T.D. patients are always deficient in some important nutrients. Providing complete supplements as a back-up system can make a big difference in achieving better health.

## Potassium

- Essential for normal heart function
- Essential for circulation
- Essential for preventing edema

## Vitamins A and D combination

- Helps mucus membranes
- Maintains bone health
- Provides back-up system for patients with a weak and malfunctioning immune system
- Important for good eye health

## Vitamin E d-alpha tocopherol

When buying vitamin E it is important to know that d-alpha is a natural product, while dl-alpha is a synthetic form of vitamin E. While vitamin E d-alpha is slightly more expensive, it alone provides the needed protection. This cannot be said for the cheaper but less effective synthetic product. To repeat:

D-alpha = natural; dl-alpha = synthetic. ***The following is a complete listing of the many important functions of vitamin E in the human body. Canadian cardiologists Wilfred Shute, M.D. and his brother Evan Shute, M.D. have given the world a wonderful gift with their vitamin E research. The knowledge, gained from their work, not only can save a person's life during a heart attack or prevent damage from a stroke, but certainly could add years of quality life. The d-alpha form is a member of the vitamin E complex

- Its specific function aids the heart and blood
- Oxygenates the blood. Its oxygenating action helps all C.T.D. patients who suffer from blood vessels spasms, which occur in Raynaud's phenomenon, Raynaud's disease and Buerger's disease
- Prevent internal clotting
- Acts as a natural blood thinner
- Provides the mechanism to help blood coagulation when it exits the body; (for instance: bleeding injuries; surgeries; tooth extraction)
- Vitamin E prevents liberation of hemoglobin from red blood cells
- Aids in the utilization of fatty acids
- Helps the heart
- Is essential for reproduction
- Is an important anti-oxidant
- Is an essential natural vasodilator
- Is a natural anti-coagulant and not only prevents blood clots, but also helps to dissolve fresh clots
- In the mixed tocopherol form it is especially effective as an anti-oxidant and combined with vitamins A, ascorbic acid and the mineral selenium, it forms a highly effective barrier against cancer cell formation
- Vitamin E protects the lungs from ozone pollution. When vitamin E levels are low in human cells the lungs can

suffer injury from ozone inhalation. The usual symptoms of ozone toxicity are upper respiratory tract infections, headaches and chest pains (Ref. Better Nutrition, 10/89, p.8. and "The Complete Updated Vitamin E Book" by Dr. W. Shute, M.D.)

- Vitamin E naturally keeps the blood at the correct viscosity
- Vitamin E prevents sludging and clotting, but at the same time prevents blood from becoming too thin. This is of special importance during and after surgery to prevent blood clots
- When exiting the body through a fresh wound, vitamin E helps the blood to immediately coagulate and close the wound against bacteria and other harmful substances
- Vitamin E increases oxygen to surrounding tissue and promotes the growth of new tissue; this speeds up healing and prevents ugly scars
- Vitamin E prevents the formation of excessive scar tissue (keloids)
- Vitamin E can be used to gradually eliminate existing scars
- Vitamin E is the most outstanding natural treatment for burns (Aloe Vera is equally effective)
- Vitamin E helps to heal serious abrasion injuries, where tissue has been lost down to the bone. It helps to form new tissue
- Vitamin E helps to prevent gangrene. It also can reverse gangrene (Ref. Dr. Shute's book)
- Vitamin E offers important protection against strokes caused by blood clots
- Vitamin E can be used immediately during the development of a stroke to minimize or prevent damage
- Vitamin E can be used immediately during the onset of a heart attack and could save a patient's life
- Vitamin E slowly reduces high blood pressure and thus offers protection against a stroke
- Vitamin E offers important protection against pulmonary

embolism

- Vitamin E offers important protection against venous thrombosis
- Vitamin E offers important protection against ulceration of the extremities
- Vitamin E is of enormous important to diabetic patients to prevent blindness
- Vitamin E helps to prevent the feared gangrene and ulceration in diabetic patients

## Vitamin E mixed tocopherol

- Mixed tocopherol is more specific as an anti-oxidant
- Offers protection against cancer and infection
- In contrast, the d-alpha tocopherol form is almost pharmaceutical in its effect on the blood itself and acts as a natural blood thinner inside the body; yet helps to coagulate blood on the outside

Additional comments: Doctors Wilfred Shute, M.D., Cardiologist and Evan Shute, M.D. have done incredible work with vitamin E, including the treatment of advanced gangrene. The reader is encouraged to study their book "The complete and updated vitamin E book" for more important information.

Vitamin E d-alpha tocopherol and Vitamin E mixed tocopherol are oil-soluble vitamins and should always be taken with meals which contain some fat. It should not be taken by itself with water. Oil and water do not mix.

## Zinc

- Protects the immune system
- Prevents aggressive behavior
- Prevents temper tantrums
- Prevents outright violence
- Prevents hyperactivity
- Zinc calms the mind

Additional comments: Zinc plays a great role in the

prevention of certain mental disorders provided it is supplemented in sufficient quantity. A deficiency in zinc results in a high copper level; it is the excess copper which causes a truly astonishing variety of mental problems (see above) and may explain the abnormally high incidence of child and spousal abuse in many homes.

## Glucosamine sulphate

- This form is much more easily assimilated than for instance Glucosamine Chondroitin or shark cartilage. It is therefore of great importance to C.T.D. patients.
- Also benefits Osteoarthritis and R.A. patients
- Repairs and rebuilds damaged tissues
- Repairs and rebuilds damaged cartilage
- Has pain relieving properties as good as and without the side effects of Tylenol or similar medication
- Dr. Michael T. Murray, N.D. states that "500 mg of Glucosamine Sulphate should be taken three times daily". This researcher pointed out that an unexpected yet very welcome benefit is "pain relief".

## M.S.M (Methylsulfonylmethane)

- Controls pain in connective tissue disease
- Helps to restore impaired tendon tissue
- Helps to restore impaired ligament tissue
- Helps to restore impaired muscle tissue

## Garlic

- Has powerful action against the toxins released by yeast fungi
- Acts equally as a powerful and natural intestinal antibiotic which prevents the build-up of dangerous toxins in the intestinal tract
- Combined with acidophilus, garlic provides important help to patients with Candida Albican and other yeast-fungal infections

- Several anti-fungal combinations are available at health food stores

## S.O.D (Superoxide Dismutase)

- Helps to improve circulation
- Helps to counteract blood vessel spasms, which are a major problem in C.T.D. patients suffering from Raynaud's phenomenon. Blood vessel spasms can cause intense pain, but also can lead to "dry gangrene" if not corrected. SOD therefore plays a very important and protective role in regaining some balance

## B6 (Pyridoxine

- Important nutrient for collagen production
- Important anti-oxidant
- Essential for lubrication of tendons
- Carpal tunnel syndrome, bursitis and tendinitis are all B6 deficiency symptoms
- Helps to prevent plaque build-up in the arteries
- A diet high in animal fats can deplete B6 reserves and is believed to contribute to arterial blockages

## CoenzymeQ10

- This nutrient is essential to cell life
- Has been identified and utilized in Japan and Europe as a major heart nutrient
- Helps prevent congestive heart failure
- Helps to improve existing congestive heart failure
- Helps prevent premature aging of cells
- Important anti-oxidant
- Q10, combined with ascorbic acid, vitamin E, selenium, B6 and various carotoid nutrients is of great value to the immune system
- Essential for normal circulation
- Q10, combined with vitamin E, ascorbic acid, S.O.D and

D.M.G is of special importance to Raynaud's phenomenon patients.

### B1 (Thiamine)

- Helps to counteract numbness and tingling sensations
- Helps to treat and prevent other neurological problems
- Helps to strengthen a weak heart
- Helps to overcome shortness of breath

### B12

- Treats and prevents "neuralgia-type" pains and is used by holistic therapists for the prevention and treatment of "trigeminal neuralgia" of the face and skull and neuralgia of the sacrum
- B12 helps to stabilize a weak heart and is of great importance to anyone with cardiac problems

### Mag. Phos. (Tissue salt #8)

- This tissue salt is used by naturopathic physicians to treat or prevent "neuralgia-type" symptoms
- Tissue salts Mag. Phos., Ferr. Phos., Nat. Mur. and Silicea are all important for connective tissue disease patients

# Author's Personal Supplement Program used for the completely natural treatment of Mixed Connective Tissue Disease with symptoms of SLE, Sjoegren's and Raynaud's phenomenon

- ¼ tsp. ascorbic acid crystals dissolved in glass of water. Rinse mouth afterwards to avoid acid causing harm to tooth enamel
- Three 500 mg Natrol Ester C with Bioflavonoids with each meal
- One 125 mg DMG sublingual with each meal.; more during active blood vessel spasms
- One 24% Ginkgo Biloba three times daily for acute conditions; twice otherwise
- One 1200 mg Bromelain once daily for maintenance. Three times daily during active "arteritis" or "synovitis" flare-ups
- Two acidophilus capsules for Candida flare-ups; one for maintenance
- One magnesium citrate 500 mg once daily to support kidneys, reduce stress and pain
- Mezotrace mineral supplement (see instructions on container)
- One Evening Primrose oil capsule three times daily (during flare-ups)

- One 100 mg B-complex with each meal
- Two 99 mg potassium tablets (consult pharmacist if taking certain medications)
- One 10,000 IU vitamin A plus 400 IU vitamin D capsule. Once daily
- One 400 IU vitamin E d-alpha tocopherol with each meal (please observe cautions stated earlier)
- One 30 mg zinc picolinate three times daily during flare-ups; twice daily otherwise
- 500 mg Glucosamine sulphate three times daily during flare-ups
- Two MSM tablets. Increase when acute pain
- One garlic tablet daily; or one clove of fresh garlic daily
- SOD taken AM and evening only
- B6 100 mg three times daily
- B1 100 mg three times daily as needed
- One 100 mg CoenzymeQ10 four times daily during first 6 months; when symptoms subside reduce to three times daily for another 6 months. When symptoms are much improved, reduce to 60 mg three times daily

Dosages and frequency depend on severity and frequency of symptoms, and age and weight of patient. Patients must adjust dosages to their individual needs. Supplements are taken with breakfast, lunch and dinner unless specified otherwise. ***Readers will undoubtedly have their own story to tell, their own pains and frustration to talk about. But, each can take a brave step forward and make a commitment to find out everything available in research and printed matter about their illness. Naturopathic physicians, reputable herbalists and health food store counselors can offer valuable help regarding product choices. ***This book could offer hope, since it not only discusses all the symptoms C.T.D. patients suffer and current medical treatment, but also offers many natural therapy solutions to ease the pain and help repair the damage. Patients can choose from natural vasodilators, natural anti-inflammatory substances and natural antibiotic substances. And they will find many other helpful suggestions to support their weakened or inflamed body, to rebuild health, and slowly but surely reverse some of the conditions causing so much discomfort. ***Alternative medicine works slowly. Patients cannot expect quick results, but can expect to be rewarded with increased "quality of life". By using supplements and herbs consistently they provide the tools needed to normalize body function. It takes time and patience; sometimes it takes many months before an improvement can be seen. But isn't it worth it? Help is here! Why not give it a try?

The author wishes to share the following affirmation which has brought great comfort and much improvement in her own battle with connective tissue disease

"Every cell of my body is filled with God's healing energy"

# Chapter V
# What is Connective Tissue?

## What is Collagen?

## And why is Ascorbic Acid so important?

Connective tissue consists of many different types of tissues; each performing different jobs. Connective tissue keeps soft organs in place, such as the lungs and stomach. It forms a sac-like structure which surrounds and holds the organ securely in place; or it provides strong, fibrous connections made from muscle to bone or bone to bone. ***Connective tissues are combination tissues, which are made up of water, protein, salts and carbohydrates and which form a gelatin-like substance. This substance surrounds each cell and each fiber.

These are the kind of cells found in connective tissue:

- White cells, which act in a defensive and protective manner
- Plasma cells, which produce "antibodies"
- Fat cells
- Fibroblast cells which make fibers

- The products of mast cells are capable of altering blood flow

All connective tissues, except hard cartilage, contain:

- Nerves
- Blood vessels

## The fibers are made of:

- Protein collagen, a very tough white substance
- Protein elastin, a yellowish elastic and flexible substance

## Areolar tissue

- A rather loose tissue which surrounds blood vessels, nerves and muscles with a protective sheath
- Both collagen and elastin fibers make up these rather soft and quite flexible tissues; this type of connective tissue holds organs like the spleen, stomach and liver in place inside the body

## Tendon tissue

- This tissue is made of much denser materials than Areolar connective tissues. Tendon tissues have great strength, because they are made up of tightly constructed collagen fibers.
- Tendon tissues connect muscles to bones

## Ligament tissue

- Ligament connective tissues consist mostly of collagen fibers
- Main function of ligament tissue is to connect bone to bone
- Without ligaments an arm, elbow or knee joint could not remain stable
- Ligaments are strong and supple. They enable us to walk, bend, stretch and give us the ability to perform very heavy

work, such as lifting or straining against heavy loads

## Cartilage tissue

- Soft cartilage provides a temporary skeletal support for the unborn fetus
- Once hardened, it becomes very dense and very tough and looks different from all other tissues because of its translucent white color
- Cartilage becomes ossified and hardens into bone, once minerals are made available to the growing tissue
- Most of the bones develop out of "rods" or "blocks" of cartilage connective tissue

## In adults we find these types of cartilage tissues:

- In the outer ear and the epiglottis we find a very elastic type, which contains collagen and much elastin
- In the human spine we find a fibrous type of cartilage, less elastin, but very tightly bundled collagen fibers. Spinal disks are made of this combination cartilage
- Hyaline cartilage is a clear and hard tissue. It is bluish in color and provides the articular cartilage
- Once developed and hardened, cartilage does not contain nerves or blood vessels, but contains many tiny channels

## What is Collagen?

Collagen is a body protein. It makes up about one third of the body's protein content and is needed for normal connective tissue health. ***Collagen is the main structural element from which blood vessels, teeth, bones and connective tissues are formed. ***Collagen acts like a glue that holds the cells of all tissues together. ***In the author's opinion, the combination of certain "abnormal factors" contribute to the development of connective tissue diseases. Each combination may result in characteristic symptoms.

### Abnormal factors may be:

- Inferior quality collagen
- Deficient collagen
- Abnormal collagen
- Insufficient collagen

### The production and synthesis of collagen depends on ascorbic acid

- Without ascorbic acid there cannot be collagen production
- When there is too little ascorbic acid available, body tissues become defective and structurally weak
- Ascorbic acid is also needed for self-repair and self-maintenance of all tissues, including the vascular vessels
- Ascorbic acid is needed for the maintenance of already present collagen
- Sufficient ascorbic is needed during the development of the embryo to provide the fetus with structurally perfect collagen protein. This need for optimum levels of ascorbic acid will continue for the rest of a person's life
- Depleted or sub-marginal ascorbic acid levels lead to a terrible illness called "scurvy"
- The majority of American citizens have low levels of ascorbic acid.. These sub-marginal levels are not adequate to produce and maintain optimal high-strength collagen over long periods of time. Defective connective tissue is the result. This can lead to all kinds of serious illnesses
- At the present time Americans obtain only a fraction of the needed ascorbic acid from their daily food intake. The human body has a huge need for this nutrient and was able in ancient times to get what it needed by eating fresh food stuff in large quantities
- All mammals, with the exception of "humans, apes and guinea pigs", produce and store ascorbic acid in the liver. During the evolution of mammals, a defective gene occurred in these three mammal categories which led to

the absence of a single enzyme. It is this enzyme which mammals need to make and store ascorbic acid in the liver. But, because this particular enzyme is missing in humans, the only way we can get enough ascorbic acid is through the food we consume.

- The modern diet does not come even close to providing sufficient amounts of this nutrient. There is never enough. On the contrary "a chronic state of deficiency exists in all humans, which makes us vulnerable to bacterial, viral and fungal diseases. This deficiency cannot be overcome, unless supplements or extremely high amounts of fresh food stuff are taken on a daily basis
- Irvin Stone, in his remarkable early book on vitamin C (ascorbic acid) presents convincing evidence, that all rheumatic diseases (connective tissue diseases) are directly linked to life-long sub-marginal ascorbic acid levels. In a nutshell... Ascorbic acid is an essential nutrient. If we don't get enough we will eventually become ill.
- Even ancient people died prematurely because of ascorbic acid and other nutrient deficiencies. Exhumed mummies for instance, show evidence of osteoporosis due to lack of calcium. Early man died young, and many did not survive infancy because of nutrient deficiencies.
- In contrast modern people have a much larger variety of food to choose from than their ancestors; yet they rely mainly on cooked or otherwise altered and nutritionally inferior food. As a direct result they develop all kinds of chronic diseases and can reach old age only with the help of many medications, surgeries and other medical help.

## Ascorbic acid can easily be inactivated or destroyed by

- Oral birth control pills
- Steroids. Ironically steroids prescribed by medical physicians for connective tissue disease symptoms inactivate what little ascorbic acid is in the body and allows the disease to get worse while fighting pain symptoms

- Anticoagulants
- Alcohol
- Analgesics
- Anti-depressant medications
- Aspirin

## Other important things to know about ascorbic acid

- Sulfa drugs and Diabinase may not be as effective when combined with ascorbic acid. One researcher stated that during pregnancy no more than 500 mg ascorbic acid should be taken daily to avoid having the infant become dependent on high amounts in the mother's blood, but then develops scurvy after birth. The author has not found any other research substantiating this claim, but leaves the choice of supplementation with the individual.
- On the positive side other researchers claim that ascorbic acid increases the action and potency of antibiotics when taken together

## What benefits do optimum levels of ascorbic acid provide?

- Wounds heal faster
- Toxic metals such as cadmium, lead and arsenic are quickly neutralized through the detoxifying action of ascorbic acid
- Many other toxic substances such as carbon monoxide are equally neutralized
- Allergies to chemical poisons can be avoided by maintaining optimum ascorbic acid levels
- Radiation poisoning can be overcome
- Viral, bacterial and fungal diseases cannot develop in the presence of mega-levels of ascorbic acid
- Optimum levels offer very strong protection against diseases such as cancer, A.I.D.S., Viral Hepatitis A, B and C and Infectious Mononucleosis
- Connective tissue (collagen) diseases could be prevented

by maintaining mega-levels of ascorbic acid.

### What about recommended dosages?

- It is generally recommended that a 140 lb. healthy person requires a minimum of 5,000 mg ascorbic acid daily to maintain optimum cell levels. If this amount cannot be provided through completely fresh and raw food stuff, then supplements should be taken
- Another researcher also lists the needs for ascorbic with 70 mg per kilogram of body weight. 1 kg equals roughly 2 US pounds. A person weighing 140 lbs. therefore would require 70 mg x 70 kg = 4,900 mg. Both researchers therefore agree on about 5,000 mg for maintenance

### This dosage should be increased however, when

- A person is much heavier than the average 140 lbs
- A person is chronically ill or experiences an acute illness
- Inherited weaknesses are known and must be addressed constantly (as in C.T.D.) through consistent ascorbic acid supplementation
- When exposure to internal and external environmental poisons are a factor
- When chronic or temporary acute high stress are depleting the adrenal gland ascorbic acid levels. Linus Pauling and Irvin Stone, both famous vitamin C researchers, agree on at least 10-12,000 mg daily taken in many divided dosages. This much ascorbic acid is best taken and assimilated in many smaller dosages throughout the day and always with some food to avoid irritation to the stomach lining. Many leading brands are available today which either have a low or neutral ph and which can be taken without irritating the stomach.

### Emergency situations which require an instant high ascorbic acid dose:

- Bee stings or other insect stings which cause an allergic

reaction. Ascorbic acid has "anti-histamine" properties and can be used until medical help arrives
- Acute high fever illness
- Poisoning
- Snake bite or the bite of other poisonous animals

When medical emergency help is unavailable a little ascorbic acid placed under the tongue every 15 minutes is an effective aid to the adrenal glands and could help avoid shock

## Which ascorbic acid supplements are most effective?

- Esterified ascorbic (known as Ester C) is the most effective. This form has been naturally chelated, bonded to minerals such as calcium, magnesium, potassium, zinc or sodium and has a neutral ph, which helps to avoid stomach irritation
- Ester C is usually sold as a complete supplement containing the entire complex of Bioflavonoids, rutin and other complex nutrients. This combination offers important added protection for blood vessel walls
- Many research projects have demonstrated that the level of ascorbic acid in white blood cells rises four times higher when the Ester form is used. Using Ester C therefore gives the immune system a tremendous boost
- Tests have shown that only one third of Ester C is excreted in the urine, while regular ascorbic acid is excreted in much higher amounts
- Another interesting fact about Ester C is that it is absorbed into the blood four times faster and remains in the cells much longer than regular ascorbic acid
- Most companies name their product "Ester C" rather than "Ester ascorbic acid".

## What else needs to be considered?

- Very high amounts of ascorbic acid are needed for acute and serious illnesses, such as "Infectious Mononucleosis",

"Viral Hepatitis", "A.I.D.S.", "Scurvy", "Poisoning" and "Connective Tissue Diseases". If a cooperative physician can be found, high levels of this nutrient are most effective when administered intravenously for immediate utilization

A basic rule...

The sicker the patient, the more ascorbic acid is needed. In the cases listed it may mean the difference between life and death to use the fastest way to get ascorbic acid into the blood stream

## Choices of administering ascorbic acid in acute illness or other emergencies:

- #1 choice = IV
- #2 choice = parenteral feeding
- #3 choice = high dosage injections
- #4 choice = high dosage tablets, powder or crystals of ascorbic acid

## For emergencies, when an IV, parenteral feedings or injections are unavailable:

- Use Ester C in many hourly dosages. Begin with 1,000 mg hourly, until loose bowels or excessive gas occurs. If and when that happens, it means that saturation level has been achieved for the time being. It must be remembered how much was used during a 24 hour period.
- For the next 48 hours use 1,000 mg less. If during these 48 hours diarrhea still occurs, dosage must be reduced again by 1,000 mg. Then take first 1,000 mg dosage early; wait 4 hours and then begin to take hourly dosages throughout the day. Adjust according to personal emergency. Bowels may stay soft, but should not be watery
- Be aware, that different products may have different dosages per unit. For instance, one company might provide 1,250 mg per ¼ teaspoon, while another provides only 1,000 mg per ¼ teaspoon. Read instructions carefully.

- Storage is important. Ascorbic acid must be kept in a dark container in a cool cabinet or refrigerator. It must never be exposed to heat, sunlight and air

## For emergencies in babies

Please, consult your medical or naturopathic physician. If help is not available use your best judgment regarding dosages. For instance, if the needed dosage for a healthy 140 lb. person is 5,000 mg daily, then a 25 lb. toddler would need roughly 1,000 mg daily through combined food and supplement intake, but more in case of severe illness or an emergency. Ascorbic acid powder or crystals can easily be stirred into juice. If the baby does not accept a spoon or glass, then the mixture can be administered with an eye dropper by releasing a couple of drops directly under the tongue. The fluid will be absorbed this way through the saliva. Pay attention to the bowels and adjust accordingly.

It is a well-known fact that low ascorbic acid levels do not always produce the obvious scurvy symptoms but still cause major changes in those metabolic processes, in which ascorbic acid is involved.

## Metabolic processes in which ascorbic acid is involved:

- Ensures calcium and phosphorus storage; vital for connective tissue
- Supports the adrenal glands; adrenals produce natural Cortisone
- Enhances vitamin E action
- Enhances the action of the entire B vitamin complex
- Increases conversion of bile acids
- Enhances iron absorption

## Why is ascorbic acid so important to the patient with connective tissue disease?

- It protects the calcium-phosphorus storage. Both nutrients are very important for bones, ligaments, tendons, muscles

and other connective tissue
- It carries oxygen to connective tissue cells
- It contributes to quick wound healing
- It is needed for healthy bones
- It is needed for healthy cartilage
- It is important as a muscle builder
- It is essential for collagen formation
- It is essential for the growth and repair of body tissue cells, gums, blood vessels, bones and teeth
- It provides important protection against viral, bacterial and fungal infections

## What are the symptoms of scurvy?

### Physical scurvy symptoms in adults:

- Capillary fragility—small blood vessels burst, seeping blood into surrounding tissue; this is seen in "spider veins"
- Petechia—small dot-sized hemorrhages into the skin or mucus membranes in patients with certain chronic diseases, or a fever which involves the entire body
- Ecchymosis—a bruise, caused by bleeding under the skin; this is also called "subcutaneous bleeding"
- Follicular hyperkeratosis—a skin overgrowth which occurs especially on the buttocks and legs
- Anemia
- Loss of appetite
- Anorexia—complete disinterest in food
- Limb and joint pain which frequently affects the knee
- Pallor and paleness
- Extreme weakness
- Bleeding and swollen gums
- Constant tooth decay
- Loose teeth
- Lethargy
- Severe lassitude, fatigue and weakness. Patient is tired all the time

- Insomnia
- Poor wound healing
- Chronic low back pain
- Hair loss
- Pronounced gastro-intestinal disorders
- Constant colds and sinus problems
- Frequent bouts with gout
- Functional impairment of joints
- Anatomical changes of joints; for instance affecting the ability to bend fingers
- Ocular hemorrhages in the bulbar conjunctiva
- Hemorrhages under the periosteum, the thin tissue which encases and surrounds bones. This is frequently preceded by itching. When the patient scratches the itchy area a sudden pain is felt and the hemorrhage occurs
- Severe ascorbic acid deficiency predisposes patient to "Rheumatic Fever"
- Severe ascorbic acid deficiency frequently produces "Tuberculosis"
- Coronary thrombosis—the majority of patients are grossly deficient in ascorbic acid
- Liver damage
- Very sensitive to heat
- Cancer

## Psychological scurvy symptoms in adults

- Hypochondria
- Hysteria
- Irritability
- Depression
- Schizophrenia
- Memory loss
- Senile dementia—premature

### Common scurvy symptoms in children

- Painful swelling in legs
- Diarrhea
- Vomiting and other gastric upsets
- Frequent fevers

### Common sub-scurvy symptoms which precede clinical scurvy and should be seen as a warning sign

- Functional impairment of joints; tenderness
- Loss of appetite off and on
- Fatigue
- Borderline anemia
- Frequent tooth decay
- Frequent bleeding of gum tissue
- Lassitude
- Complaints of all kinds of health problems
- Slightly depressed
- Chronic low back pain
- Some hair loss
- Spontaneous bruising
- Occasional nose bleeds
- Growing pains
- Slow healing bruises
- Gastro-intestinal problems
- Slow healing fractures
- Frequent colds and sinus problems
- Beginning of a cataract
- Tendency towards gout
- Arthritic lesions
- Bothered by prickly heat

# The role of ascorbic acid in connective tissue diseases arthritis and rheumatism

- Both rheumatoid arthritis and osteoarthritis, rheumatism and related rheumatic conditions are considered connective tissue (collagen) diseases, establishing a definite involvement of the "collagen protein" in all these diseases
- High levels of ascorbic acid are essential to help the body to synthesize high quality collagen and to maintain this quality
- Collagen makes up about one third of the body's protein
- When an ascorbic acid deficiency occurs, either collagen protein synthesis stops altogether or shows up as poor quality protein. This results in weakened and abnormal tissues
- An ascorbic acid deficiency creates negative bone and joint effects which fall into the category of "clinical scurvy"
- Abnormalities in the collagen protein are the reason for crippling deformities associated with rheumatic disease and other congenital connective tissue defects
- Rinehart and co-workers wrote in their 1930-1938 research

that "deficiencies of ascorbic acid plus an infection are responsible for the rheumatoid process". It was also stated that "rheumatic fever is caused by a major ascorbic acid deficiency". Other contributing factors are malnutrition, the effect of climatic changes, stress factors, how old a patient is at the onset of the disease, and geographical distribution

- The research further states that there are "symptomatic similarities between rheumatic fever and latent scurvy"
- Vast numbers of later experiments were done with ascorbic acid, only to be discontinued because the researchers could not duplicate the wonderful results of earlier research. Reason for their failure was that they were trying to simply correct a nutritional deficiency, using very small amounts of ascorbic acid, when they should have been treating a serious disease (scurvy) with mega-doses of ascorbic acid. Just raising the blood level to normal simply was not enough. The blood level must reach megascorbic levels in the very ill person to achieve an improvement or cure.

To summarize…

Ascorbic acid must be provided at megascorbic levels to have a definite therapeutic effect on connective tissue diseases. Several researchers suggested that in acute or chronic cases even six to ten grams daily given by IV or orally were successful in providing anti-rheumatic activity. In one such case the researcher listed a patient suffering from "rheumatic fever" receiving up to ten grams (10,000 mg) of ascorbic acid daily. taken in divided dosages throughout the day. Rapid improvement followed, with a c complete recovery in three to four weeks. The suggestion is being made to provide higher amounts if they are tolerated well. In all critical cases ascorbic acid should be given by IV whenever possible.

# Chapter VI
# A private study involving eleven connective tissue disease patients

Based on the many different symptoms connective tissue disease patients experience and which may involve several organs, gland structures, muscles, tendons, ligaments and other tissues, the decision was made to develop a questionnaire and find out, what all these sick people have in common. The author developed this questionnaire over a period of several months and finally placed a small ad in the local newspaper inviting C.T.D. patients to meet as a group. About twenty very sick folks showed up. Hannelore identified herself to the group as an experienced holistic nutrition practitioner and researcher, but also as a C.T.D. patient. She discussed her own multiple symptoms and then asked the participants to talk about their diagnosis, their symptoms and prescribed medications. She spoke about her understanding of the illness and her strong belief that natural medicine could do much to help. Each visitor was handed the questionnaire and asked to answer all questions. Eleven of the twenty elected to do so. This group was invited back for a second meeting during which the survey results were discussed. In addition, each participant received personalized information, which nutrients, herbs or other natural substance or therapy might be of help in that patient's particular situation.

The following subjects were covered in the study:

- Childhood diseases
- Adult illnesses
- Family health patterns, such as diabetes, heart disease, mental disease etc.
- Inherited weaknesses
- Immunizations; any reaction to them
- Nutritional habits in childhood and adult years
- Blood test history (e.g. high lipids, high blood sugar, anemia, etc.)
- Diagnostic procedures used, such as medical, chiropractic, acupuncture, naturopathic, reflexology and iris diagnosis
- Present medications used
- Known allergies
- Hair analysis data
- Heavy metal or chemical toxicity
- Information about child-bearing years in women
- History of glandular function
- History of infections
- Past surgeries
- History of stress
- Mental health history
- Nervous system history and spinal health
- General body pain history, including headaches
- Blood sugar problems
- Urinary system function
- Reproductive system function
- Respiratory system function
- Digestive system function
- Circulatory system function
- Problems with bones, muscles, ligaments and tendons
- Skin, nail and hair changes—a history of...

- Health of teeth, mouth, ears and eyes
- History of body temperature (e.g. chronically low temperature or constant fevers)
- History of unusual body odors and their significance

## Study results

Comparing the "major symptoms these eleven study participants share" can shed some light on the subject of connective tissue (collagen) disease. Since all study subjects were females and most of them middle aged and older, this study is neither conclusive nor representative of other patients. But some very interesting facts emerged:

- All eleven had chicken pox in childhood = viral
- Seven have chronic Candida Albicans = fungal
- Seven have/had chronic fungal infections of finger and toe nails = fungal
- Seven have/had repeated episodes of warts, cankers and fever blisters = viral
- All eleven list viral and fungal infections as recurring problems
- All eleven reported at least two or more overlapping symptoms (e.g. Raynaud's and Sjoegren's, or Lupus and Raynaud's)
- Nine were inoculated with small pox vaccine = viral
- Nine reported heavy antibiotic use throughout their lives
- Over half of the study participants are now allergic to fermented food items, mold, mildew, fungi, penicillin and similar medicine
- Questions about surgery revealed that nine had their tonsils removed and six had appendectomies. (the tonsils and appendix are part of the immune defense system and the removal of this lymph tissue weakens the entire immune system)
- Family patterns revealed a very high incidence of heart disease, cancer and a variety of mental problems; all indicative of substantial and chronic nutrient deficiencies

- All but one share a poor nutritional start in life, beginning with the fact that most were not breast fed (poor immune system start). Only half eat home-cooked meals as adults
- High refined sugar use is apparent in this study. Ascorbic acid, chromium, magnesium and trace element deficiencies are common in such individuals. Especially an ascorbic acid and magnesium-manganese deficiency can greatly contribute to the development of connective tissue disease
- Based on the information the eleven participants provided one has to conclude that at no point in their life did their bodies receive optimum nutrition
- Chronic stress due to the presence of chronic illness further depletes any nutrient reserves and contributes to the development of depression and/or suicidal thoughts. The study revealed such tendencies
- Half of the participants reported salt and/or sugar cravings. This is a clear sign that the mineral metabolism is not normal. For instance, heavy use of candies, soda pop and chocolate can lead to a substantial magnesium deficiency, which in turn can contribute to suicidal tendencies
- Ovary and thyroid problems were reported by most of the eleven participants (nutritional deficiencies can impair glandular function)
- Digestive disturbances in the form of alternating constipation and loose bowels affected nine patients and can be explained with the presence of Candida Albicans
- Seven participants reported blood sugar problems within their family units
- Dizziness and palpitations were common occurrences in six study participants. In the author's opinion contracted neck muscles can affect vertebral positioning and misalign cranial sutures and cause a multitude of seemingly senseless symptoms. A misaligned cervical spine can result in severe dizziness, palpitations and various ear noises.
- Numbness and tingling in the extremities or on the main

body, face, nose and lips were common symptoms

- Feelings of paralysis of the epiglottis, tongue and esophagus were also reported
- Feelings of bugs crawling through the hair or inside the ears are malfunctions of the nervous system. These symptoms were also reported by several participants. These symptoms are caused by substantial nutrient deficiencies and can be corrected through specific supplementation (see nutrient section) Six of the eleven participants reported these unusual and scary sensations and further commented that doctors or family would not take them seriously or wrote them off as being "neurotic".
- Other unusual feelings reported were that the brain suddenly would slow down; words would not come easily; words within a sentence would get mixed up; or one word would be made part of another, creating a totally different word; or not being able to complete a sentence or form a complete thought. Studying the incredible effects of B-vitamin deficiencies can enlighten the reader and explain these unusual symptoms
- Erratic behavior of body temperatures was reported by seven participants. They reported feeling really cold one minute and then suddenly feel a rush of heat (blood vessel spasms) throughout their bodies; and/or experience sudden and short periods of excessive perspiration. Others did not sweat at all; a definite sign of a substantial ascorbic acid deficiency
- Only one participant experienced beginning gangrene symptoms. However, Raynaud's phenomenon produces blood vessel spasms which not only shut down circulation to wherever the spasms are felt, but can cause severe tissue damage because of lack of oxygen. Addressing the problem of blood vessel spasms and preventing gangrene has to the number one priority of C.T.D. patients. Essential nutrients must be provided to regain normal tissue function
- Since all C.T.D. patients suffer from various muscle,

ligament, tendon or synovial problems, the underlying multi-mineral and ascorbic acid deficiencies must be corrected

- Miscellaneous complaints, such as hang nails (lack of Silica), dry mouth and gritty eyes (lack of ascorbic acid), crusty build-up inside nostrils (lack of B-vitamins) or the development of a fatty apron in the lower abdomen (explained by Chinese medicine as a hormonal problem and by the author as a deficiency in tissue salt #12 Silicea) are symptoms reported by several of the study participants
- Several participants reported vision disturbances, heavy floaters, light flashes and slight problems with double vision. Ascorbic acid plays a very important role in these occurrences
- Major body pains were reported by all eleven participants and require a major nutrient approach to restore the integrity of blood vessels, nerve tissues, bones, muscles, ligaments, and tendon and synovial tissues
- Grand mal and petit mal seizures were not experienced by any of the study participants but were reported as having occurred within their family units. Holistic researchers link seizure activity to a substantial magnesium deficiency
- Many participants reported frequent night urination. Often this problem is caused by consistent bladder and kidney infections or inflammations, which can be caused by repeated antibiotic treatments and resulting Candida Albicans fungal infections
- Several participants reported shortness of breath and a severe vice-like pain in the rib cage and/or inner wall of the upper abdominal cavity. This symptom severely interferes with breathing and sufficient oxygen uptake

## Progress report

### Final comments by the author

In 1988 I suffered a major health breakdown which I

eventually self-diagnosed as "mixed connective tissue disease". I experienced many confusing symptoms, which initially were overwhelming because they involved so many different body organs and functions. I spent over 30 years in practice as a holistic practitioner and therefore approached my problem with the mind set that my body is capable of correcting itself, once I understand the underlying causes. But how could one find the cause of malfunction of so many body parts? It took years of patience and persistence, but also complete faith in "universal energy" to slowly regain control of my body. And I have proven to myself that alternative therapy methods can and will lead to a healthier life and state of mind. The commitment to a totally holistic approach to my own health problems certainly has prolonged my life in a positive way. ***This book is based on the wonderful research of literally hundreds of earnest and many well-known researchers. Among them are many men from the medical field who have contributed greatly to my understanding of the human body. I will provide a "suggested reading" list to honor some of my mentors. No, I did not graduate from a famous medical school. My degree is a specialized degree in holistic nutrition. It may mean nothing to most medical physicians; but I can say that in the end the only thing that counts is knowledge, experience and honesty. It is my most sincere wish that the reader finds help and hope through this book. ***I can summarize the major improvements in my health achieved with only holistic medicine as follows:

- The initial symptoms of severe circulation shut-downs caused by blood vessel spasms have been reduced to a minimum and signs of gangrene were reversed through specific nutrients. I avoid exposure to anything with strong vibrations (e.g. chain saw; rock music; any strongly vibrating hand tools or household gadget; long rides in an automobile or airplane)
- Fungal infection flare-ups and pain are being kept to a minimum with a careful diet which limits food containing

yeast, fermented products or fungi in any form. I have eliminated all sugar products. If a flare-up occurs the appropriate natural medicines (Acidophilus, garlic, Lysine and Tea tree oil) are immediately used. I also use an herbal anti-fungal tincture, which is very effective

- I reduced my stress level. Sleep is peaceful and productive. I awaken refreshed and full of energy
- Mood problems are totally absent now
- Crying spells are absent now. In earlier years I discovered that my thyroid did not function normally and added Kelp to my daily nutrient intake. Kelp provides iodine which in turn aids thyroid function
- My general attitude is optimistic
- May mind is clear and productive
- Low blood sugar episodes are very rare now; in earlier years they made me feel spacey, flaky and disconnected
- Pain in skull muscles, neck muscles and contracture pains in rib cage are improved by at least 80% and occur less often
- Pain and tissue weakness in ankle and wrist joints is completely corrected now through consistent ascorbic acid supplementation
- Problems with occasional edema, high blood pressure and some kidney discomfort occur only during acute yeast-fungus flare-ups and subside when the crisis is over. Acute flare-ups are quite rare now
- Swelling of fingers and hands and slowness of hand and finger movements has been corrected
- Sore mouth and bleeding gums are no longer a problem

It is my opinion that chronic yeast-fungal infections and consistent low ascorbic acid levels cause most of the symptoms connective tissue disease patients' experience. While patients may be predisposed genetically the disease may never develop, until unrelenting mental stress, substantial nutrient deficiencies or toxic substances overwhelm all body defenses. Yeast/fungal infections produce many toxins. ***The reader will remember the significance of ascorbic acid in maintaining normal adrenal gland function and the importance of many other nutrients which help to maintain normal cell function. Through my own experimentation I have found a strong relationship between yeast-fungal infections and the incidence of lung congestion, bronchial congestion, edema, bloating, shortness of breath, constant low grade to moderately high fevers and much severe pain. I discovered that each time the symptoms of yeast-fungal infections (itching, weeping yeast lesions in groin, vagina, and underarms and sometimes in fatty folds of the body) improved, so did the pain, the fevers, congestion, edema and high blood pressure. What I learned is this: Without eliminating this major problem first the body simply cannot heal itself. By supporting the body through very specific nutrients, herbs or other natural substances, the opportunity is provided to regain normal function.

Each patient must carefully examine his/her health history and make the needed adjustments to regain health and productivity and with that quality of life. It takes a lot of self-discipline and hard work, but it can be done. There is hope!

Affirmation

"Every cell of my body is filled with God' healing energy"

# Index

Acidophilus 130, 162, 188, 244, 249, 297
adrenal glands 12, 59, 65, 76, 80, 88, 91, 97, 215, 218, 219, 237, 275, 278
exhaustion 88, 97
affirmation 10, 264
alcohol 271
alkaline gut 81, 199, 215
allergies 272
ANA test 107, 154
anemia 110, 283, 288
cerebral 89, 130, 207
Anorexia 280
anti-bacterial 188
natural 17, 18, 55, 57, 92, 125, 156, 185, 188, 190, 193, 196, 204, 207, 210, 211, 212, 213, 217, 244
antibiotics 17, 24, 52, 97, 162, 272
natural 9, 12, 13, 14, 17, 18, 23, 24, 54, 55, 58, 60, 74, 79, 80, 82, 83, 84, 88, 89, 90, 91, 92, 119, 124, 125, 126, 127, 128, 130, 131, 145, 160, 176, 177, 182, 184, 190, 191, 193,

194, 195, 198, 199, 200, 206, 209, 210, 212, 214, 217, 218, 221, 243, 244, 245, 247, 249, 252, 253, 254, 255, 256, 259, 262, 263, 264, 278, 287, 288, 297, 300
anticoagulants 271
anti-depressant 53
anti-fungal 18, 24, 125, 188, 189, 259, 298
arterial spasms 14, 40
Arteriosclerosis 149
Arteritis 193
arthritic lesions 283
artificial tears 52
ascorbic acid 18, 54, 55, 58, 80, 83, 86, 88, 95, 97, 98, 123, 151, 152, 164, 188, 201, 203, 205, 215, 218, 220, 222, 227, 230, 231, 232, 233, 234, 235, 236, 237, 239, 240, 242, 246, 247, 251, 254, 260, 262, 268, 269, 270, 271, 272, 273, 274, 275, 276, 277, 278, 279, 281, 284, 285, 286, 291, 294, 298, 299
Osteoarthritis 200, 201, 258
Rheumatism 200, 201
Rheumatoid arthritis 200, 201
submarginal levels 242
Ascorbic acid 54, 55, 58, 59, 90, 91, 128, 164, 181, 185, 186, 188, 190, 191, 193, 198, 199, 202, 205, 211, 212, 214, 225, 233, 235, 236, 241, 242, 247, 269, 270, 271, 274, 277, 278, 285, 291, 295
Bartholins glands 44, 48
birth control pill 106
bladder 18, 98, 104, 125, 134, 135, 136, 137, 138, 139, 140, 295
blindness 47, 233, 234, 256
blood coagulation 253
blood pressure 41, 52, 53, 57, 66, 73, 74, 78, 84, 89, 90, 97, 114, 119, 128, 159, 197, 200, 204, 208, 209, 210, 218, 219, 239, 240, 256, 298, 300
blood sugar 234, 248, 249, 288, 292, 298
blood tests 16, 42, 97, 169, 180

blood vessels 14, 36, 61, 62, 63, 65, 66, 67, 73, 77, 80, 84, 87, 94, 137, 142, 145, 147, 148, 149, 150, 153, 154, 155, 156, 158, 164, 166, 169, 204, 208, 210, 240, 243, 253, 266, 268, 279, 280, 295
weakness 48, 65, 102, 144, 151, 168, 169, 170, 172, 174, 175, 176, 179, 280, 298
spasms 28, 29, 32, 33, 36, 37, 41, 42, 67, 148, 154, 155, 162, 166, 197, 200, 208, 209, 253, 259, 262, 294, 297
body temperature 87, 289
bowel 11, 183
brain 24, 104, 121, 125, 129, 144, 204, 207, 208, 222, 223, 226, 242, 248, 293
breast 230
bruising 114, 283
burning sensation 41
bursitis 129, 194, 259
Calcinosis 61, 66, 145
cancer 52, 159, 230, 282
Candida albicans 139
capillary damage 34
cardiovascular 18, 125, 183, 243
carpal tunnel 129
cartilage 84, 147, 169, 193, 225, 226, 258, 265, 267, 268, 279
cavities 12, 47
Cayenne 91, 164, 188, 209
central nervous system 94, 104
chills 39
cholesterol 205, 207, 208, 209, 210, 239, 241
Chromium picolinate 248
circulation 6, 15, 22, 27, 41, 66, 67, 74, 77, 81, 89, 90, 91, 130, 153, 157, 164, 176, 177, 179, 196, 197, 205, 206, 207, 208, 209, 212, 222, 248, 252, 259, 260, 294, 297
circulatory system
dizzy 242
edema 41, 114, 116, 210, 234, 252, 298, 299, 300

peripheral 27, 41, 81, 89, 90, 164, 166, 197, 207, 208, 40, 289
CoenzymeQ10 54, 59, 74, 90, 123, 130, 162, 178, 179, 181, 191, 197, 205, 211, 222, 231, 260, 263
colds 159, 281, 283
collagen 14, 18, 61, 62, 83, 85, 128, 164, 165, 186, 201, 202, 239, 241, 247, 259, 266, 267, 268, 269, 273, 279, 284, 290
confusion 48
connective tissue 6, 8, 13, 14, 16, 17, 18, 20, 22, 27, 29, 45, 48, 49, 51, 63, 79, 85, 86, 89, 93, 98, 107, 119, 126, 133, 134, 146, 147, 148, 149, 151, 165, 168, 169, 171, 180, 182, 184, 185, 186, 193, 201, 204, 212, 213, 247, 251, 252, 258, 261, 264, 265, 266, 267, 268, 269, 270, 271, 278, 279, 284, 285, 287, 290, 291, 296, 299
essential fatty acids 121, 185, 212
manganese 90, 185, 198, 225
mineral supplement 128, 131, 196, 226, 246, 262
MSM 91, 177, 184, 193, 194, 198, 199, 200, 263
nutrients 14, 17, 22, 24, 43, 44, 65, 66, 77, 85, 86, 87, 89, 123, 127, 131, 133, 134, 145, 147, 154, 176, 184, 185, 191, 204, 214, 217, 218, 220, 224, 227, 228, 230, 233, 242, 247, 250, 252, 260, 275, 279, 288, 294, 297, 299, 300
tissue salts 131
cornea 56, 237
corneal epithelium 56, 237
cramps 196, 197, 209
crying spells 40, 298
dementia 222, 248, 282
depression 79, 104, 112, 114, 220, 222, 291
Dermatomyositis 17, 20, 64, 150, 168, 170, 172, 178
diabetes 52
diabetic retinopathy 55
diaphragm 38, 82, 116
diarrhea 101, 282
digestive system 41, 289

bloating 7, 41, 72, 144, 299
constipation 72, 101, 170, 292
esophagus 7, 29, 38, 41, 56, 62, 66, 67, 69, 72, 74, 84, 85, 151, 236, 293
hiatus hernia 38
loose bowels 41, 277, 292
reflux 41, 67, 72, 74
Discoid Lupus Erythematosus 17, 85, 111, 112, 113
Discoid rash 111
DMG 89, 188, 190, 191, 247, 262
dry eyes 45
dry skin 34
ear noises 292
ears 29, 30, 46, 95, 100, 167, 289, 293
Endocarditis 103, 107
epiglottis 39, 267, 293
eyes 7, 15, 28, 42, 44, 47, 50, 52, 55, 56, 215, 233, 235, 236, 237, 289, 294
corneal ulcers 47, 235
dry 34, 52, 53, 54, 55, 56, 57, 74, 233
eye ball 30
floaters 295
glaucoma 78, 112, 182, 234
retina 56, 144, 235, 236, 237
facial bones 30
facial erythema 100
fatigue 46, 99, 105, 143, 282
feet 32, 33, 35, 39, 40, 64, 66, 81, 130, 147, 151, 153, 155, 156, 166, 208, 215, 216
fetus 116, 267, 269
fevers 11, 23, 101, 282, 289, 299
Fibromyalgia 17, 49, 180, 250
Fibrosis 69
fingers 27, 34, 39, 62, 66, 67, 99, 143, 153, 155, 157, 166, 167, 227, 281, 299
fluid retention 38, 41, 140

fractures 283
gangrene 14, 22, 35, 85, 89, 102, 144, 145, 148, 150, 151, 153, 154, 155, 158, 161, 163, 166, 204, 206, 248, 255, 256, 259, 294, 297
garlic 188, 190, 191, 193, 210, 217, 244, 258
gastritis 42
Ginkgo Biloba 89, 123, 130, 164, 193, 197, 198, 207, 208, 211, 212, 218, 222, 232, 248, 262
Alzheimer's 222, 248
arterial leg disease 208
blood flow 89, 144, 148, 149, 150, 151, 161, 162, 167, 204, 205, 207, 208, 210, 222, 265
glands 11, 30, 33, 43, 44, 45, 46, 47, 49, 50, 51, 54, 76, 77, 80, 83, 87, 91, 101, 195, 196, 199, 215, 218
Glucosamine sulphate 92, 177, 199, 200, 224, 225, 226, 257, 263
gout 281, 283
growing pains 283
gums 46, 49, 64, 74, 279, 280, 299
Hamstring muscle 33
hand movements 39
Hawthorn berry 162, 208
headaches 7, 29, 65, 144, 159, 200, 254, 289
hemorrhages 239, 242, 280, 281
hepatitis 205
hoarseness 46, 175
honey comb 56
hyperkeratosis 280
hypochondria 282
hysteria 282
immune system 12, 45, 47, 63, 86, 90, 93, 96, 123, 128, 129, 142, 148, 163, 176, 178, 182, 191, 208, 225, 226, 248, 252, 257, 260, 275, 291
immunosuppressive drugs 51
Inclusion Myositis 168, 174
infant 272

infection 38, 52, 72, 85, 107, 114, 136, 139, 140, 142, 201, 256, 284, 297
infections 17, 18, 20, 23, 38, 77, 78, 86, 87, 96, 98, 102, 104, 105, 106, 115, 125, 130, 162, 182, 215, 244, 249, 254, 259, 279, 289, 290, 295, 299
Infectious Mononucleosis 273, 276
inflammation 23, 30, 45, 68, 81, 84, 102, 103, 104, 114, 115, 136, 138, 139, 140, 142, 154, 168, 169, 176, 177, 181, 193, 194, 195, 197, 199, 213
insomnia 114, 217
intestinal flora 11, 92, 123, 130, 162, 191, 249
Iridology 16
iron 224
irritability 104, 282
Irvin Stone 234, 270, 274
jaw 7, 29
Juvenile Myositis 168, 175
Kelp 80, 83, 91, 163, 186, 218, 226, 227, 231, 298
kidneys 48, 84, 94, 103, 117
abnormalities 42, 103, 105, 119
hematuria 103
malfunction 43, 62, 66, 71, 76, 77, 86, 87, 116, 136, 214, 296
nephritis 104, 136, 140
proteinuria 103
renal infarction 104, 136
renal thrombosis 131
stone 135
toxicity 86, 98, 254, 288
lassitude 280
legs 29, 32, 33, 36, 39, 41, 81, 102, 130, 143, 151, 152, 161, 206, 207, 227, 280, 282
lens 56, 237
lethargy 280
ligaments 14, 32, 87, 147, 151, 169, 193, 196, 198, 224, 225, 267, 279, 287, 289, 295

Linus Pauling 16, 165, 186, 274
lips 39, 40, 57, 58, 69, 114, 292
liver 48, 94, 109, 282
lungs 38, 65, 66, 72, 84, 90, 102, 115, 144, 161, 206, 239, 254, 265
degeneration 239
lymph 30, 76, 77, 81, 82, 84, 90, 195, 196, 199, 291
magnesium 59, 129, 181, 193, 196, 199, 220, 222, 227, 246, 250, 251, 262, 275, 291, 292, 295
memory loss 208, 222
mental problems 105, 257, 291
mind 125, 222, 257, 296, 298
mixed connective tissue disease 27, 180
Morphea 68
muscle tissue 32, 33, 158, 248, 258
muscles 7, 11, 14, 28, 30, 31, 32, 33, 35, 36, 37, 38, 65, 66, 69, 70, 101, 147, 148, 149, 151, 152, 169, 170, 175, 193, 196, 197, 198, 220, 221, 224, 266, 279, 287, 289, 292, 295, 298
Myopathies 168
nails 11, 33, 143, 212, 290, 294
neck 7, 33, 34, 37, 50, 69, 95, 99, 100, 111, 117, 152, 292, 298
nerves 27, 40, 76, 149, 221, 224, 266, 268
nervous system 39, 289
neurotic 12, 106, 109, 293
nose 27, 40, 47, 56, 69, 95, 100, 111, 166, 167, 172, 205, 283, 292
NSAD 183
numbness 15, 26, 40, 67, 144, 150, 186, 227, 251, 260
nutrients 1, 2, 3, 4
ovaries 218
pain 6, 7, 8, 15, 18, 20, 21, 23, 27, 28, 29, 30, 31, 32, 33, 36, 37, 38, 41, 49, 55, 56, 58, 64, 65, 76, 87, 91, 92, 93, 99, 100, 101, 102, 112, 114, 117, 125, 126, 129, 134, 135, 136, 137, 143, 144, 149, 150, 151, 152, 157, 172, 175, 176, 177, 178,

181, 193, 194, 195, 196, 198, 199, 200, 206, 208, 209, 214, 219, 228, 236, 249, 250, 251, 258, 259, 262, 263, 264, 271, 280, 281, 283, 289, 295, 297, 299
ankle 26, 32, 298
arm 8, 26, 27, 37, 69, 121, 130, 267
bones 36, 37, 65, 69, 147, 152, 196, 198, 224, 266, 267, 268, 279, 281, 289, 295
cerebellum 39
face 26, 27, 33, 34, 37, 39, 64, 66, 67, 70, 94, 99, 111, 114, 261, 292
finger tips 27, 157
kidney 18, 38, 51, 59, 65, 71, 90, 102, 103, 109, 115, 116, 117, 122, 123, 124, 125, 131, 134, 135, 136, 137, 138, 139, 140, 214, 228, 295, 298
leg6, 22, 26, 27, 36, 69, 121, 163, 197, 200, 204, 208, 209
neuralgia 100, 129, 236
rib cage 32, 36, 38, 102, 152, 295, 298
TMJ temporal mandibular joint 66
palpitations 292
pancreas 40, 48
Pantothenic acid 80, 86, 214, 216, 251
paralysis 39, 242, 293
parenteral feeding 276
pelvis 33
penicillin 11, 12, 97, 188, 290
perspiration 77, 294
Petechia 143, 280
phosphorus 278, 279
photosensitivity 100
pituitary 43, 218, 237
pneumonia 103
Polymyositis 17, 20, 64, 150, 168, 169, 170, 174, 180
Prednisone 78, 114, 116, 170, 172, 182
prickly heat 283
Primary Sjoegren's syndrome 44
pulmonary embolism 256

pulmonary hypertension 149
radiation 231, 273
rashes 23, 33, 99, 100, 102, 112, 115, 133, 143, 175, 178
butterfly 95, 100, 101, 111
cutaneous 93, 94, 111, 145
discoid 17, 85, 93, 94, 111, 112, 113
Raynaud's disease 17, 20, 49, 147, 166, 167, 204, 248, 253
Raynaud's phenomenon 17, 20, 22, 27, 29, 31, 61, 67, 68, 80, 100, 101, 103, 128, 145, 147, 148, 149, 151, 154, 155, 158, 159, 160, 161, 167, 176, 177, 180, 204, 236, 248, 253, 259, 260, 262, 294
reflexology 288
Reproductive system 38, 289
bleeding 29, 46, 74, 79, 114, 205, 240, 253, 280, 283, 299
cramps 41
iregular menses 101
ovary 292
respiratory system 38, 289
fungal infections 24, 98, 295, 299
rheumatic fever 57, 84, 89, 128, 201, 202, 285, 286
rheumatoid arthritis 45, 107, 284
sacrum 35, 81, 82, 179, 261
scars 95, 104, 111, 112, 146, 154, 155, 255
Schizophrenia 222, 282
sciatic nerve 33
Sclerodactyly 62, 67
Scleroderma 6, 17, 20, 22, 37, 49, 61, 63, 64, 67, 68, 69, 71, 72, 73, 74, 75, 76, 77, 79, 80, 85, 86, 88, 89, 91, 107, 145, 149, 159, 165, 168, 180, 195, 199, 208, 212
CREST 61, 62, 66
diffuse sysemic sclerosis 61
telangiectasis 62, 67
Sjoegren's syndrome 32, 44, 45, 49, 50, 51, 55, 64, 74, 88, 107, 149, 168, 233, 236

skin 18, 23, 33, 34, 39, 46, 47, 59, 61, 62, 65, 66, 67, 68, 69, 70, 73, 74, 76, 77, 81, 82, 84, 87, 94, 95, 102, 111, 113, 128, 130, 131, 133, 145, 147, 148, 150, 151, 154, 155, 157, 169, 172, 182, 188, 212, 213, 214, 227, 280
changes 78
discolorations 214
hardened areas 85
sores 99, 130, 213
tender 28, 34, 46
vitiligo 11, 33, 100, 213, 214
skull 7, 28, 29, 32, 33, 37, 152, 261, 298
sleep 15, 40, 47, 121, 197, 217, 220
Slippery Elm 56, 84, 238
small pox 290
SOD 89, 129, 259, 263
speech 39
sphincter 134
stomach 7, 42, 66, 85, 102, 114, 175, 195, 246, 265, 266, 274, 275
spine 31, 32, 82, 267, 292
cervical 292
lumbar 136
sacrum 35
thoracic 31
sternum 32, 36, 38
steroids 51, 116, 182, 271
stress 9, 11, 12, 20, 24, 42, 71, 77, 80, 86, 88, 91, 96, 122, 123, 124, 158, 183, 201, 220, 222, 227, 240, 249, 250, 262, 274, 285, 289, 291, 298, 299
stroke 242
sugar cravings 23, 292
suicidal 222, 291, 292
sun exposure 93, 113, 158
surgery 144, 149, 153, 254, 290
synovial membranes 224

Systemic Lupus Erythematosus 17, 45, 49, 64, 93, 149, 168, 176
aggression 223
alopecia 101
anemia 102, 105, 280
blood clots 102, 128, 131, 133, 161, 206, 243, 254, 255
bruises 117, 143, 283
butterfly rash 101
convulsions 117
digestive problems 7, 41
drug induced lupus 93, 95, 119
dyspnea 103
high fever 195, 274
kidney problems 65, 71, 102, 115, 228
leg ulcers 102, 163
mouth sores 109
myocarditis 103
neurological problems 18, 104, 125, 176, 260
oral ulcers 57, 100
parotid gland 100
pericardititis 103, 239
scurvy 18, 83, 97, 185, 201, 202, 239, 240, 269, 272, 278, 279, 282, 284, 285
seizures 97, 105, 144, 295
urinary tract problems 134, 137
vasculitis 17, 20, 48, 102, 142, 143, 144, 145, 146
Systemic Sclerosis 17, 61, 64, 65
Tachycardia 103
taste 53, 54, 57, 152
teeth 12, 29, 64, 268, 279, 280, 289
decay 29, 280, 283
loose 280
tendinitis 259
tendons 14, 32, 33, 36, 66, 87, 147, 151, 169, 193, 196, 198, 224, 225, 259, 279, 287, 289
thirst 57

throat 29, 30, 39, 56, 79, 238
Thymus 190
thyroid 12, 43, 65, 76, 80, 83, 85, 86, 91, 107, 163, 187, 218, 219, 292, 298
tingling sensations 179, 260
toes 35
tongue 31, 39
Tuberculosis 281
urinary system 104, 228
alkaline 42, 83, 246
cystitis 135
frequent urination 38, 139
kidney 71, 102, 109, 115, 134, 135, 139, 140
mucus in urine 141
nephritis 144
renal vein thrombosis 136
ureteritis 136, 140
urethritis 136
uterus 219
vagina 44, 48, 299
dryness 46, 48, 50, 51, 55, 57, 58, 218
lubrication 15, 46, 48, 57, 59, 259
vaginal tissue 57
vascular vessels 269
vasodilators 18, 73, 82, 125, 176, 209, 264
vasospasms 128, 154, 155, 156, 158, 163, 166, 187
venous thrombosis 256
vibrations 27, 39, 155, 297
viral Hepatitis 273, 276
vision 47, 55, 65, 144, 233, 295
vitamin E 55, 57, 84, 85, 122, 128, 145, 203, 204, 214, 222, 231, 241, 243, 252, 253, 254, 255, 256, 260, 262, 279
vocal cords 56
vomiting 101, 117, 282
wounds 146
healing 159

wrist 151, 298
yeast fungus 23, 41, 86
zinc 43, 57, 223, 231, 233, 234, 257, 263, 275

# Suggested Reading

"Psycho Nutrition"
by Carlton Fredericks, Ph.D.
"Health & Light"
by John N. Ott
"Mental and Elemental Nutrients"
by Carl C. Pfeiffer, Ph.D., M.D.
"The Encyclopedia of Common Diseases"
By the staff of Prevention Magazine
"Life Extension"
by Durk Person and Sandy Shaw
"Brain Allergies—The Psychonutrient Connection"
by William H. Philpott, M.D. and Dwight K. Kalita, Ph.D.
"Complete Book of Minerals and Complete Book of Vitamins"
by J.I. Rodale and staff
"Nutrition against Disease"
by Dr. Roger J. Williams
"The Pulse Test—easy allergy detection
by Arthur F. Coca, M.D.
"Zinc and other Micro-Nutrients"

by. Carl C. Pfeiffer, Ph.D., M.D.
"The doctor who looked at hands"
by John M. Ellis, M.D.
"Ortho-Molecular Nutrition"
by Abram Hoffer, Ph.D., M.D. and Morton Walker, D.P.M.
"Cancer and its Nutritional Therapies"
by Richard A. Passwater, M.D.
"The Rejuvenation Vitamin"
by Carlson Wade
"Folk Medicine"
by D.C. Jarvis, M.D.
"Complete ... Updated Vitamin E Book"
by Wilfrid E. Shute, M.D.
"The Healing Factor—Vitamin C against Disease"
by Irwin Stone, Dr. Linus Pauling and Dr. Albert Szent Gyorgyi
"Adrenal Syndrome"
by G.E. Poesnecker, N.D., D.C.
"Prescription for Nutrition Healing"
by James F. Balch, M.D. and Phyllis A. Balch, C.N.C.
"Disease"
by Nurse's Reference Library
"Feed Your Kids Right"
by Lendon Smith, M.D.
"The Human Brain"
by Isaac Asimov
"The Human Body"
by Isaac Asimov
"The Edgar Cayce Handbook for Health Through Drugless Therapy"
by Harold J. Reilly, D.Ph.T., D.S. and Ruth Hagy Brod
"P.D.R. People's Desk Reference—Traditional Herbal Formulas I and II"
by Joseph Montague
"The Herb Book"
by John B. Lust, N.D., D.B.M.

"Back to Eden"
by Jethro Kloss, herbalist
"Schwester Bernardines Heilkraeuter und Hausmittelbuch"
by Orbis Verlag Gmbh., Muenchen, Germany, 1988

# About the author

Hannelore Helbing-Sheafe was born and raised in Germany, came to this country in 1959 and married Harry P. Sheafe, a well-known chiropractic physician in the Pacific Northwest. Hannelore pursued her own career in the holistic field as a Master Reflexologist, licensed Massage Therapist and Holistic Nutrition Counselor and Researcher, while raising daughters Susanne, Karen and Christa. She received her Doctorate in nutrition in 1984. She published a successful first book "Reflexology, The Ultimate Health Connection" in 1987. This was used as the textbook for all workshops and classes she taught in the Northwest, including the prestigious Evergreen State College in Olympia, Washington. She has an intense interest in the relationship between nutrition and disease. During her 30-hear practice, her patients received therapy for symptoms presented, along with nutritional guidelines to address the causes. Out of the vast research material compiled for her practice, a second book emerged in 1988, "The Bare Facts" which explains underlying causes of, and presents natural treatment options for most known skin diseases, hair and nail problems. Many other titles have followed since, including those on the topics of connective tissue diseases, Lyme disease and Trigeminal Neuralgia.

Made in the USA
Lexington, KY
04 October 2011